SHOULDERS OF GIANTS

A Facial Surgeon's
prescriptions for life's dilemmas

SHOULDERS
OF GIANTS

Coach "Bear" Bryant's
"price of victory"
is re-examined by
E. Gaylon McCollough, MD, FACS

ALBRIGHT & COMPANY   1986
HUNTSVILLE

"Shoulders of Giants" is about as inspirational a collection of thoughts as I have seen anywhere. There is no lack of guts in this book. Dr. McCollough tells it like it is."

Thomas W. Rhodes, Attorney
Smith, Gambrell & Russell
Atlanta, Georgia

Library of Congress Catalog Card Number 86-071697
ISBN: 0-932919-04-9

Typesetting by Bruce Graphics, Inc.
Birmingham, AL

Author's Note

For my conferrer, partner, and wife of 22 years —
my *best* friend — Susan Nomberg McCollough

For my parents, Olin and Gladys McCollough, whose love, guidance,
and faith helped *me* believe I could do "it". . .

For our children, Sted and Chanee — be the best that
you can be. . .

And. . .

For being an American, and having the chance to say and do
as we choose. . .

———————

Because I believe in what they are about, the author's royalties of
Shoulders of Giants shall be donated to the following institutions:

> —Enterprise High School, Enterprise, Alabama

> —The Bryant Hall of Honor, The University of
> Alabama

> —John Croyle's Big Oak Ranches for abandoned boys
> and girls

> —The American Academy of Facial Plastic and
> Reconstructive Surgery, Inc.'s Educational
> Foundation

E. Gaylon McCollough, MD

Acknowledgements

My sincere thanks goes out to the following people who believed in *Shoulders of Giants* and the message it is intended to deliver.

Dr. Joab Thomas, President, The University of Alabama, Tuscaloosa, Alabama

Thomas W. Rhodes, Attorney, Smith, Gambrell & Russell, Atlanta, Georgia

Father Timothy Hill, John Carroll High School, Birmingham, Alabama

Carolyn Perkins, Tuscaloosa, Alabama

Dr. Jack R. Anderson, New Orleans, Louisiana

Dr. Richard C. Webster, Boston, Massachusetts

Dr. Bill Beeson, Indianapolis, Indiana

Fred Russell, Vice-President, the *Nashville Banner,* Nashville, Tennessee

Paul Bryant Jr., Tuscaloosa, Alabama

. . . . .

A *special* debt of gratitude is owed to

Alf Van Hoose, sports editor, *The Birmingham News* for his assistance and confidence,

to

Rosemary Metcalf and the rest of my secretarial staff,

to

Wayne Atcheson, Director of Sports Information, The University of Alabama,

to

Charles Nesbitt, *The Birmingham News,*

And finally . . . to

Millford Kelly, my English teacher at Enterprise High School, who taught me how to express my thoughts with pen and ink.

Table of Contents

Continued

Contents, continued

PART IV
"WHAT MEN DARE DO"

PART V
A LOOK AT MEDICINE AND THE LAW

PART VI
THE MASTER PLAN

Comments from reviewers...

If a picture is worth a thousands words, a real life experience accurately related should be worth a thousand theoretical models.

Dr. McCollough has described in vivid and intimate detail, the impact on his life of a few great leaders— one in particular, Paul W. Bryant. *Shoulders of Giants* is also an excellent study of the role and significance of competitive sports in developing strength of character.

> Dr. Joab L. Thomas
> President
> The University of Alabama

Viktor Frankl [*Man's Search for Meaning*] a prisoner at Auschwitz and other Nazi camps claims that one finds meaning in life in three different ways; by doing a deed, by experiencing a value, and by suffering. Dr. McCollough highlights these three ways with openness and sincerity. Reading his book enriched my life—it certainly can enrich yours.

> Father Timothy "Ted" Hill
> John Carroll High School
> Birmingham, Alabama

"I found *Shoulders of Giants* to be both practical and inspiring. Dr. McCollough's revealing account of the challenges forced upon him by those protecting *turf* has much to teach each of us. Gaylon talks of "giants"—he's emerging as one himself."

> Richard C. Webster, M.D.
> Plastic Surgeon
> Boston, Massachusetts

"*Shoulders of Giants* provides the reader with insight into the inner strength necessary for championship performance in any arena. It is unique, thought provoking, and stimulating—essential reading for anyone who strives to reach his fullest potential."

Bill Beeson, M.D.
Indianapolis, Indiana

"Dr. McCollough has succeeded by applying the lessons learned in football in the remainder of his life; young people would do well to emulate this uncommon man."

Jack R. Anderson, M.D.
New Orleans, Louisiana

"I appreciate the feelings toward Papa conveyed in *Shoulders of Giants* . . . Gaylon's account of the selection and hiring of Ray Perkins as head coach is especially informative . . ."

Paul W. Bryant, Jr.
Tuscaloosa, Alabama

"*Shoulders of Giants* reveals how knowledge and experience gained from others helped Gaylon face life's dilemmas. In my opinion, he now has giant shoulders upon which young men and women can stand."

Carolyn Perkins
Tuscaloosa, Alabama

Gaylon McCollough was a center, a very good one, under one of the master teachers of young men and his art—Paul Bryant.

Football centers have a special analytical advantage. At work they view from an unconventional posture, giving them, overall, a truly balanced look.

The future Dr. McCollough's experiences under Bryant honed a perceptive gift which has continued to flower, first in surgery, now in a book.

You are guaranteed a conscientious reminder that what we *are* is not by chance, but by choice.

Alf Van Hoose
Sports Editor
The Birmingham News

*"Destiny is not a matter of chance,
it is a matter of choice;
it is not a thing to be waited for,
it is a thing to be achieved."*
                    William Jennings Bryan

A Course of Excellence

On the wall of my study hangs a treasured picture of a giant upon whose shoulders many have climbed. The following message was inscribed when it was given to me:

> *"To Dr. Gaylon McCollough,*
> *Thanks for being a great player, a great doctor,*
> *a class person and my friend.*
>
> *If you believe in yourself and have dedication*
> *and pride—and never quit, you'll be a winner.*
> *The price of victory is high—but so are the*
> *rewards.*

Paul 'Bear' Bryant"
(12/16/81)

Coach Bryant was one of the great men whose principles provided the basis of this book. He, and all the others to whom the credit is owed, demonstrated that self-analysis, self-esteem, self-control, and work are the keys to achieving a destiny of excellence.

The best preparation for the future is an understanding of the past. Almost everything has been said before—somewhere, sometime, somehow. My objective in writing this book is to examine what has been said (and done) *again*. I have re-examined it from the perspective of both a student and a teacher using syllogistic reasoning. In doing so, it should have *new* meaning for the person who believes that he can and should do something meaningful with his life.

Chances, choices, and challenges are the necessary ingredients for discovering who one is and what he is destined to do. There are many individuals with more intelligence, wisdom, talent and courage than I.

*I am only one, but I am one. I cannot do
everything, but I can do something.
What I can do, I should do, and with the
help of God, I will do it!*[1]

While being confronted with the many distractions of a 20th century society, it is difficult to stay on a course of excellence. The price of victory *is* high. If we are willing to pay the price, the rewards shall surely be worth the effort.

SHOULDERS OF GIANTS is one man's analysis of the factors which lie at the roots of both excellence and mediocrity. It is also a book about life, not just my own, but about mankind. Within these pages are found syllogistic prescriptions for life's dilemmas. As the pages unfold, each person who reads them should come face to face with some aspect of his or her own life and recognize that each of us has much in common. Change the names, dates, and places, and my dilemmas become like your own. Hopefully, the conclusions I reached through deductive reasoning will provide insight and help resolve yours, and ours.

What we can do we should do, and with God's help, we can transcend mediocrity. A course of excellence is a matter of choice.

Let me tell you how I see things—from the "shoulders of giants."[2]

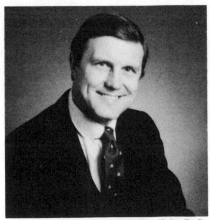

E. Gaylon McCollough, M.D. F.A.C.S.

---

[1]Everett Hale, *The Rebirth of America* p. 233.
[2]Lucan, Didacus Stelle, *The Civil War,* A.D. 39-65.

Introduction

CHANCES, CHOICES AND CHALLENGES

"It's a funny thing about life;
If you refuse to accept anything
but the best,
You very often get it"[1]

If we want to come face to face with the person who controls our destiny, we need only to look into a mirror. Who we are and what we become is based upon how we respond to opportunity, achievement, and failure. Self-esteem and self-control can only follow self-analysis.

The American Heritage Dictionary defines "syllogism" as "a form of deductive reasoning consisting of a major premise, a minor premise and a conclusion."

This book and my philosophy of life have evolved from the following syllogism.

If,

> great men and women (giants) view the world from a position of knowledge, wisdom, and courage (major premise);

And,

> mortals are capable of seeing clearly (minor premise);

---

[1]Somerset Maugham, *Motivational Quotes* p. 2.

1

Then,

> mortals who choose to climb upon the shoulders of great
> men and women (giants) should be able to see what the
> giants see. (conclusion)

The choice is between mediocrity and excellence. The climb to excellence is not an easy expedition. One can expect opposition, criticism, and distractions. The journey to mediocrity, on the other hand, is short, smooth and simple. It's easy to be one of the crowd, or to fail.

If the choice is to pursue a course of excellence, we can rise to greater heights by climbing upon the shoulders of giants. Perched there, we are allowed to see things more distant and more clearly. This revelation is not due to the greatness of our own size nor the keenness of our own eyes, but because the great men and women who are proven giants in their fields of endeavors have borne us aloft by their knowledge, preserved us with their courage, and sustained us with their wisdom.

From this elevated position, we can examine the virtues, values and valor which epitomize excellence. We can also diagnose the elements of deference, despondency, and delinquency which characterize mediocrity or failure.

Each time we adopt the behavior patterns and thought processes of role models, a type of reincarnation occurs. Through us, then our children and our children's children, proven policies and standards of excellence of wise and excellent individuals live over and over again.

There are no new problems—just different times, places, people, and circumstances.

Champions learn how to overcome adversity. "He was good at what he did . . . he achieved success in an unconventional manner . . . they tried to mar his reputation . . ." It's a predictable scenario for those who stick their heads above the crowd. Horace, the philosopher, said, "Adversity has the effect of eliciting talents which in prosperous times would have lain dormant."

Throughout their lives achievers are confronted with *gut-checks* which makes them either *bitter* or *better.* All dilemmas have been solved at least once. Where do we find the answers? When we seek solutions to today's challenges, we should remember that, "The value of short sayings of wise and excellent men is beyond estimate. . ."[2]

Throughout both my life and this book, I have relied upon the sayings of "wise and excellent" men and women as pillars to undergird my philosophy of life. My convictions evolved from the qualities of excellence I have extracted from the great individuals of yesterday and today who I chose as role models. This book is intended to be a tribute to the giants who have allowed me to "see more clearly."

In publishing my book, at this particular time, I have taken a calculated risk. I have divulged my formula for problem solving and shared some real-life examples where the method was tested. I have laid myself bare. Some people will get ideas. That is my goal—to challenge stagnant minds, to encourage the uncertain, and to stir the rest. The things you are about to read are intended to open some eyes. After much deliberation, I became convinced that writing my book was an idea whose time had come. Lee Iacocca told his story. I gained insight through his experiences. His book helped inspire me to publish mine. Between the two, there are some similarities. There are, however, numerous differences. I decided to tell my story and let the chips fall where they may.

Why would I do such a thing? I am a student of learned men and women. I also consider myself a teacher, a medium through which knowledge passes to the next generation. In my capacity as a teacher, I feel compelled to share what I have learned, believing that each of us gains insight through the experiences of others. I did, and I hope you will.

Who is man? From whence did he come? Why does he exist? What is his destiny? We cannot understand our species without first going through an exercise of self-analysis. Before psychiatrists are allowed to practice psycho-analysis on their patients, they are required to go through the process themselves, first hand. Experience, coupled with knowledge, provides a stronger foundation for problem solving.

There is a problem faced by mankind. In mathematics, while searching for answers, we learned that a whole is the sum of its parts. What factors constitute the "parts" of our species? Each of us is a composite of both our genetics and the environment to which we have been exposed. Life is a journey through time encountering yes-

---

[2]Leo Tolstoy, *Seeds To Sow* p. 99.

terdays, todays, and tomorrows. Along the way, we are faced with dilemmas, forcing us to take alternate routes. How we handle the difficult times often dictates the difference between success and failure.

Mankind has a common origin and a common destiny, but between those extremes a fine line divides success from failure, excellence from mediocrity. In many instances, it is a matter of choice. First, man is given the opportunity to decide between good and evil. Assuming the choice is to reside on the side of good, one could develop self-esteem by devoting one's life to study and work. By doing so, one can *make* things happen for one's self. One could, however, decide to take the easy road and allow opportunities to pass by—to be a bystander in the game of life.

As our lives evolve, the characteristics of role models we select are reproduced in us, so we must be careful when choosing them. Humans are "copycats". We adopt the behavior of those with whom we mentally and physically associate. We are not only known by the company we keep, we become part of the company we choose to keep.

Share with me the deductive reasoning I used in choosing a career which best suited my abilities. I concluded that man is given the opportunity to decide whether he wishes to focus his energies on a well defined target—to go whale hunting—or to throw his net into the sea and capture whatever swims by. In the professional and business world, as well as in athletics, one chooses to become either a specialist or a generalist, to conquer a single mountain or several hills. There is a significant difference. I took a chance and became a *facial* plastic surgeon instead of a *general* plastic surgeon. It was my choice. Chances, choices, challenges, and courage are the elements from which self-control is conceived.

Along the way toward reaching my goals, it was necessary to select role models and to draw upon the wisdom of great men and women who had already worked out the solutions to many of the problems I faced. I will show how the experience gained from my years in the athletic arena was invaluable in helping me deal with the man-made obstacles which stood between me and my goals in life's game. One learns that the instant he chooses to play for one team, he immediately inherits opposition from the players and supporters of the opposing group. Not everyone is happy for the winner. It is a rude awakening. Surviving opposition is a universal problem. Unfortunately, human nature is . . . human nature.

We will look into the sometimes ruthless game of medical politics as it is played with malice in Alabama and across the U.S.A., analyzing some of the methods and motives of the players on both sides of the issues.

I want you to examine with me some of the challenges ahead for the medical profession from within and without, when physicians' problems become the public's problems. We will see what may become the destiny of health care in America.

Manhood is a mountain to be conquered. As I look back, I realize that in becoming an athlete, a husband, a father, and a facial surgeon, it has been necessary to examine my own convictions and to draw upon the wisdom of those I consider giants in order to cope with life's ups and downs. That's how one grows. That's when insight awakens. Therein lies the secret to self-control.

This book is dedicated to the giants I have known—my family, teachers, colleagues, and friends—all the great men and women of today and yesterday who have elevated the rest of us. They provided the opportunity, direction, and knowledge for me to do something meaningful.

See if you agree.

PART I
A LOOK AT MANKIND

CHAPTER 1

CHOICE BEGINS WITH A CHANCE

"Man's mind, once stretched by a new idea, never regains its original dimensions."[1]

As Pan Am flight 073 soared over Turkey, Rumania, Hungary, and Austria, I looked from the window of the large jumbo jet and reflected upon experiences of the past week. Susan and I were returning from a seminar where I had been teaching plastic surgery of the face and nose to surgeons in India. During the previous five days, my mind had been stretched to new dimensions. Borne aloft by the wings of the giant craft, the world could be viewed from a different perspective. From 50,000 feet above the ground the "big picture," can be viewed more clearly. It is as though one can look into both the past and the future. I fell into a state of deep thought.

We flew over first one country and then another. I realized that boundaries dividing one nation from another are not natural, but made by man. Mankind has allowed itself to be fragmented into political, social, economic, religious, and ideological subgroups. How did it happen? Why has it occurred? Has mankind really made mean-

---

[1]Oliver Wendell Holmes, *Motivational Quotes* p. 10.

ingful progress? Has human nature changed since Adam and Eve? Is the earth any better than it was centuries ago? During the last 100 years, technological advances have multiplied—but are we simply rediscovering what has been known for eons by other civilizations elsewhere in the universe? Could it be that life is a cycle that has no beginning or end? Is life a symphony performed over and over again by The Supreme Maestro? Are we simply the performers, new players on a permanent stage? Where does each of us fit in the time cycle?

Now is a constantly moving thing. What time it is depends upon *when* one asks the question. Every second is a sickle which divides the past from the future. Today's achievements are tomorrow's trophies. Tomorrow's trophies are yesterday's memories.

In the context of time, which is more important, yesterday, today, or tomorrow? Everything is relative. Microcosmos within macrocosmos. Man's energy represents sparkles in a vast universe searching for something to illuminate.

Had I been part of the completion of a cycle? Plastic surgery of the nose had returned to its roots. I was invited to India to teach plastic surgery of the nose to the nation that originally introduced it to the rest of the world. The first nasal plastic surgical operation was performed in India around 600 B.C. Amputation of the tip of the nose was a common type of punishment for certain domestic offenses, such as adultery. Innovative surgeons of India developed a surgical procedure whereby the nose could be reconstructed with a flap of skin from the forehead. Throughout the world, a similar procedure is still used today for some types of nasal reconstruction following cancer surgery or accidents.

During our week in India, I came to realize that a fine line exists between the civilizations of the twentieth and the fifteenth centuries. Simply stepping across the threshold of the door of the large Pan Am jumbo jet allowed us to re-enter the comfort of the modern western world. We stepped from yesterday into today. Within seconds, it seemed that we spanned five hundred years of time. Isolated areas of India enjoy twentieth century technology, education, and the basic amenities of the western world. Across the street from state-of-the-art technology, however, some Indians facing insurmountable odds live in mud and stick huts, walk around naked, and barely survive, as did their forebearers centuries ago. Where was their self-esteem?

Do they have a choice? Did they have a chance?

India is truly a country of contrast. Yesterday and today exist simultaneously, one seemingly ignoring the other, as ships passing in the night. Two distinctively different civilizations were out of phase in time—one moving forward, the other marking time. It is man's nature to search for ways to make his life better, though change may not be indicative of progress. It depends upon one's point of view.

Symbols of Excellence

In Agra, India, stands the Taj Mahal, one of the so-called seven wonders of the world. It is a majestic structure erected by a fifteenth century monarch as a monument to his beloved wife. He intended it to be a lasting symbol unlike any monument ever built. Its elegance, harmony, balance, precision, and technical detail testify that although mankind has come far in materialistic ways, it may never surpass the talents and accomplishments of architects, artists, and craftsmen of the past. In today's hurry-up world, we seem to want everything erected quickly and economically. Even "art" is produced on an assembly line basis. "Quick-fix" often replaces quality. Speed without quality is meaningless. The difference between mediocrity and excellence can be a matter of choice, or pride.

> *"People forget how fast you did a job—but they remember how well you did it."*[2]

The Taj Mahal took 20,000 craftsmen 22 years to complete. Has man since achieved such artistic excellence? We certainly have the inbred talent and ability, but today we tend to depend upon technology rather than craftsmanship. If we have the talent, tools, materials, knowledge, and ability, then, could it be a lack of motivation and pride that leads toward mediocrity? With the standards of excellence established by the masters of the past as a heritage, how do we go about reaching greater heights as students, athletes, surgeons, engineers, scientists, and artists? Achievement comes through a combination of accomplishments and failures. We build upon one, learn from the other.

---

[2]Howard W. Newton, *Motivational Quotes* p. 12.

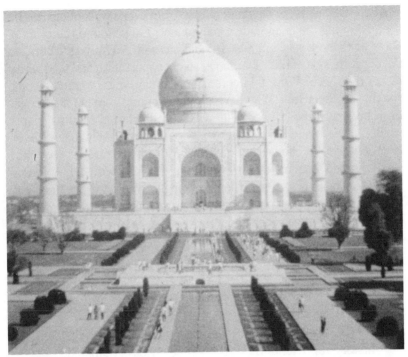

Taj Mahal

Are some given better chances than others? It seems that those who can see no other way out accept the cards life has dealt, without signs of malice. Even though famine, filth, and ambivalence surrounded the walls of The Taj, there appeared no resentment from individuals who, by chance of birth, became paupers instead of priests, beggars instead of philanthropists, laborers rather than industrialists.

Mankind needs symbols which provide identity, hope and purpose. In India, the Taj Mahal stands as a beacon in a sea of despair, symbolizing love, beauty, precision and achievement to all who see it— rich and poor, young and old, man and woman. The poet, Leer, once said, "The world can be divided into two groups of people, them that has seen (it) and them that hasn't (seen it)." The structure seems to have that kind of impact on those who appreciate it. People from all social strata are reduced to equals standing before The Taj. Great individuals seem to have this same type of effect on people. Some call it "presence." These giants either intimidate or inspire us.

At any moment, hundreds of people from every walk of life can be seen admiring this magnificent monument. Looking into the faces of some of those helpless souls, I could but ask, "Why was I born on the opposite side of this globe, in a land of opportunity and prosperity rather than here? Why, did I come into a family which wanted me and could provide for me? Why have so many opportunities for achievement been available to me? Why was I exposed to intellectual giants willing to teach and share their wisdom with me? Why have I been given chances to choose my destiny? More importantly, now that I have climbed one mountain, what am I to do with what I have learned? There is a reason for all things. When we are finished, maybe there will be some answers—prescriptions for dilemmas, both yours and mine.

Looking At The Future

Does history really repeat itself?
Syllogistically. . .

If,

      history represents the recorded behavior of mankind;
And if,

      man's instinctive behavior is inbred;
Then,

      future men shall behave as did their forebearers.

Enter a variable. Man, unlike other species, can choose to alter his behavior. Wise and excellent men and women have transcended instinctive behavior through self-control.

Insight obtained through self-analysis and courage bolstered by self-esteem allow the informed to choose excellence over mediocrity. If mankind practices self-control and makes wise choices, the face of history can be altered by following the principles of any well-conceived plastic surgical endeavor. Man's destiny can be a matter of choice.

We shall examine the parts of the master puzzle which holds the keys to the unique qualities of man and the mortgage on the planet upon which he lives.

Is it possible to predict the future? Some prophets appear to have been blessed with such a gift. On the other hand, mortals and computers can anticipate probabilities. To do so, each must first be informed of data from both the present and the past.

Knowledge is the discovery of that which already exists. Wisdom is knowing how to use it. Our future is merely a series of probabilities of how mankind will react to his options. If we understand instinctive behavior and recognize the possible events which could occur at some point in time, it may be possible to anticipate how man, as an individual or as a group, might respond to similar sets of circumstances. The psychologist might refer to this as "behavior patterns." The sociologist might consider it "mores." To Nostradamus and to John, it was a "revelation." To most of us, it is "human nature."

The Man Who Saw Tomorrow

Dr. Michell de Nostradamus, a Frenchman born in 1503, was a prophet, a man who clearly saw and recorded the future. Had he never written his prophetic *Centuries*, history would still have recorded him as one of the most outstanding French physicians who ever lived. He was, in addition to physician and prophet, a linguist, scholar, diplomat, writer, and teacher—a true "Renaissance man."

In the Biblical book of Joel, God tells His people that, "your sons and daughters shall prophesy. Your old men shall dream dreams, your young men shall see visions." Nostradamus, by record, "was the greatest of all who since Biblical ages to have given to these words the substance of fulfillment."[3]

Many people have the ability to anticipate events which might occur in the future. Certainly, some have abilities far superior to others, but there is strong evidence that each human brain has the ability to "anticipate" future events, like a computer can print out probabilities.

Nostradamus claimed that his psychic gift was inherited, but he apparently developed it, as the athlete develops his body, by pushing it beyond its current capacity. In his attic, night after night, he saw farther and farther into the future.

As his gift grew, Nostradamus, like most men of genius, felt the urge to share his visions with his fellow man. He could see destiny and felt compelled to tell the world what he saw. It was his belief that

[3]Nostradamus, *The Man Who Saw Through Time* (McCann, Farrar, Straus & Giroux, 1941), pp. XV-XVI.

a prophet cannot contradict "laws of destiny." Nostradamus said,

> *"Destiny, a man's or a nation's, is according to a divine plan . . . The prophets of Scripture did not utter to change that plan, but through perceived truth to lead men closer to God."*[4]

"That plan," I believe, is the destiny of the planet earth, not the destiny of each individual character on life's stage. We are given choices. God allows each of us to select the character we wish to play and allows us to play the role as we choose on His stage. That too, I believe, was His plan, to allow us to choose our own destiny within the rules of the game.

Nostradamus was a physician before he was a prophet. He had the vision of men and times. He saw tomorrow. Because he cared about his fellow man, he attempted to forewarn us of the events he saw. Hundreds of the "visions" he described over 400 years ago have already occurred, as he recorded them.

A physician and a prophet, Nostradamus wanted to help people. His conclusion and message to us is that a people must help themselves. All that can be done is to arouse people and to hope that wise men will take heed. One of my goals in writing this book is to arouse the mind of each person who reads these pages.

Mankind, while living within the confines of time allowed for this planet, has a destiny of choice. According to the prophecies of Nostradamus, there is a good chance that major physical changes on the earth's surface—catastrophies such as floods, earthquakes, wars, etc.—might occur at the time of the double eclipse, which will take place in the year 1999. The events described in his works are reminiscent of those described by John in the Book of Revelations, except that those of Nostradamus could have been based upon celestial phenomena derived from the scientific studies of astrology and astronomy, while John's were based upon a dream in which God revealed the events of Judgement Day to him.

Of interest is that both are identical, yet derived from different sources more than 1400 years apart—one scientific, one theological. Many have argued that scientific and divine phenomena cannot exist

---

[4]*Ibid*, p. 172.

simultaneously. If scientific or cosmic events are under the absolute direction of a Divine Intelligence, the two could be one and the same. Time will tell.

This man, Nostradamus, was a phenomenon. His works are eye-opening. Does he describe destiny or does he describe a series of probabilities based upon the predictable behavior of mankind—behavior which seems to have remained unchanged through the ages? It appears that Nostradamus saw both the stage and the actors. He named and described the behavior patterns of Hitler, Napoleon, Pasteur and Franco more than 300 years before any of them existed and accurately described the indelible mark each made in history, before it occurred. It was his conclusion that, "The fatal order of destiny is an eternal chain, forever looping on itself in cycles consistent with its own order."[5] If this is the case, was Nostradamus seeing into the future or far into a past, eons ago? Was he remembering or prophesying? Is destiny "an eternal chain...looping on itself in cycles. . .?"

That is not a question we have the ability of answering at this time. It is a problem far beyond the imagination and understanding of mortals, but we can dream and wonder. Our role is not to tamper with God's plan, but to direct our own life as He has allowed—to do the best we can during our time on earth. Our duty is to choose a destiny which makes our lives meaningful—to be the best we can be with the talents awarded us.

Follow Loaded Wagons

One of the unique qualities that separates man from the other animals is the fact that he is capable of setting a goal beyond existence—to find a *better* way of life. The pursuit of those goals is like playing a giant game—for keeps. The outcome is recorded in a record book more important than any here on earth.

We know that people can generally be divided into three groups: those that don't know (or care) what happens, those that watch things happen and those that make things happen. It is those who make things happen who become the players in life's game. Those who merely observe wonder why the players are driven to participate with such intensity. Some men play games for the sport of it—some

---

[5]*Ibid*, p. 184.

play to win. Is there a key to winning? From my observations and experiences, I believe that knowledge establishes the necessary foundation, talent and work are the tools, and commitment provides the power to open the door leading to fulfillment.

Each step involves interaction with one's fellow man—anticipating his behavior. Strategy exists both in athletics and in the game of life. Knowing the shortcomings and tendencies of the participants on both sides of any issue helps establish a winning game plan.

We can learn by two principle methods: by trial and error or by drawing upon the wisdom of those who already know some of the answers. Dr. James J. Hicks, one of my teachers, advised: "Don't follow an empty wagon around. Nothing's going to fall out of it."

I have been fortunate to walk with and behind individuals whose wagons were loaded. Along the way, I have picked up some useful bits which I have attempted to load into the pages of this book.

I would hope this soliloquy is a wagon of sorts, and that all exposed to it will benefit from my experiences, as I did.

Public Opinion

In playing the game of life, how do we know when we have won? Who is the judge of success or failure? Who or what entity evaluates us along the way? According to Mark Twain, the judge's name is public opinion. "Public opinion," he said, "is held in reverence. It settles everything. Some say it is the voice of God."[6]

In this regard, I can't agree with Twain. Public opinion is fickle. Like the wind, it can go either way. It can be changed by well-conceived advertising campaigns or rumor. Public opinion is the voice of *man*, not that of God. His voice is the same yesterday, today, and forever. The voice of man is subjected to the test of time. It endures for only as long as the memory and values of good men remain constant.

What qualifies one mortal to judge another mortal? Each man is struggling for the solutions to his own problems. An unknown author once said that man comes into the world without his consent. He leaves it against his will. When he is little, the big girls kiss him. When he is big, the little girls kiss him.

Who a man truly is and how he is perceived by others may differ.

---

[6]*Bartlett's Quotations.*

If he makes a lot of money, people may think he is dishonest. If he is poor, he's labeled a bad manager. If he needs credit, he can't get it. If he is rich, every lender wants to help him. If he is religious, he is often called a hypocrite. If he doesn't openly profess his faith, he's a sinner. If he gives to charity, it's for show. If he doesn't, he's stingy. If he is affectionate, he is a soft specimen. If he doesn't appear to care, he's a cold-hearted scrooge. If he dies young, there was a promising future for him, but if he lives to a ripe old age, he's an outdated old fogy. If he is a winner, he is a hero; but if the same man loses, he can become a scapegoat for the frustrations of those who are unable to make things happen for themselves.

How quickly public opinion can change. The world rewards winners. It usually forgets losers.

Public opinion follows trends and generally follows those who are most persuasive, not necessarily those who are most truthful. We cannot afford to put ourselves in a position of dependence upon others to determine who or what we are and can become.

In March of 1986, Susan and I judged a beauty pageant in Geneva, Alabama. Along with Betty Baggott, we selected a candidate for the National Peanut Festival in Dothan. As we interviewed the contestants, many volunteered that "peer pressure" was one of the greatest dilemmas facing America's youth. Conforming to the ways of the crowd invites mediocrity or failure.

The person who sets his own goals and standards, then sticks to them, can overcome peer pressure. That person will emerge, in the end, the victor over mediocrity. A look inward, coming face to face with one's self, may be the most important step in controlling one's destiny, self-analysis, self-esteem and self-control. Let's go back to the beginning.

The Destiny of Man

All human beings are products of both genetics and environment. Scientists still cannot agree which is the dominant factor.

In looking back at my own life, I believe that there has been a balance between genetics and environment. I'm not sure either has been dominant. Both have been crucial in providing a solid foundation upon which I could stand to develop as an athlete, a person and a facial surgeon.

This much we do know: instinctive behavior is inbred, conditioned behavior is learned. Good seeds, properly cultivated, yield good fruit. The opposite can also be true. The world contains good people and not-so-good people. Accordingly, we must learn to deal with both. We will look at examples of each that I have encountered.

Does a "good" person become "bad" because he is exposed to "bad" people, or is psychopathic behavior inbred? What are the qualities that separate good from evil, mediocrity from excellence? Is it luck?

> *"The only good luck many great men ever had was being born with the ability and determination to overcome bad luck."*[7]

Big Oak Ranch

In 1974, following the completion of an outstanding football career at The University of Alabama, John Croyle turned down a chance to play for the Dallas Cowboys. He chose, instead, to follow another dream and established a home for abandoned children.

A few months later, he found a small farm just outside Gadsden, Alabama, and his dream became a reality. The future of Big Oak Boy's Ranch was insured when John Hannah, a teammate at The University of Alabama (later an All-Pro with The New England Patriots), turned over to Croyle his play-off bonus money, $29,000.00.

Today, Big Oak is the home of boys who were either abandoned or given up by their natural parents. John Croyle and his wife, Teresa, have dedicated their lives to seeing that young men might have a chance to choose their own destiny. Unselfishly, they give their energy and time to boys that nobody wants.

Ray Perkins, one of Big Oak's most loyal supporters, recently said, "John Croyle is my hero. What he does is far more important than winning football games."

Soon, Part II of John Croyle's dream, a separate ranch for girls, will become a reality. He has a commitment from a supporter to build the first house for abandoned girls as soon as the site has been se-

---

[7]Channing Pollock, *Motivational Quotes* p. 50.

cured. Not only because he is 6'7" tall, but because of his commitment to mankind, John is a giant among mortals—a good man who has devoted his life to help young people help themselves.

Most of us are given a much better chance at home than the boys who come to Big Oak Ranch. We are born to parents who want us and want to give us every chance to make lives for ourselves. Choice begins with a chance, but there is more to life than chance. Each person deserves a chance to make decisions that will allow him to control his destiny. We should not be afraid to make decisions. The decision to attack, retreat, surrender, or simply do nothing is still a decision. Too many choose to do nothing, insuring failure. Hundreds, maybe thousands, shall prosper because John Croyle chose to devote his life to seeing that homeless children could have a chance.

Tenants On A Planet

We do not yet fully understand the delicate balance between environment and genetics, but we do know that man is unlike the other animals. He is more likely to turn on the hand that feeds him. Mark Twain said, "If you pick up a starving dog and make him prosperous, he will not bite you. That is the principal difference between a dog and a man."

I learned this lesson from a couple of the surgeons I trained. People seem to have short memories. What is it about this creature, man, that makes him different? Is it greed, envy or jealousy? If it is, how do jealousy, envy, and greed affect man's actions against his brother? Maybe one day soon, we will not only understand more about behavior and other scientific events, but will be able to affect what has sometimes been considered fate. How many years ago were the concepts of "test tube babies," embryo implantation, heart transplants, the implantation of artificial organs and joints into our bodies, or putting a man on the moon ridiculed by skeptics? Have we just begun to explore what some "civilization" somewhere in the universe has known from the beginning of time?

In March of 1986, on a trip to Bogota, Columbia, to teach plastic surgery of the nose to surgeons in South America, I was introduced to a professional photographer. She shared an unusual experience with Susan and me.

When she developed a candid snapshot she had taken of an old man strolling up a hillside, she discovered what appeared to be artifact at the top of the photograph. After several unsuccessful attempts to brush away the artifact, she decided to enlarge the photograph. To her amazement, she had captured, on film, what appeared to be an unidentified flying object. For fear of being ostracized, she told no one of her "discovery" for ten years.

The flattened cone-shaped object with its trail of spiral-shaped exhaust is clearly visible in the upper left corner of the photograph streaking across the skyline of the mountain range outside Bogota, Columbia.

As I sat there in her living room staring at the photograph of this craft, several questions leaped into my head. Was I seeing a photographic trick or a piece of the master puzzle? If it was real, where did it come from? Where was it going? What was its mission? To whom did it belong? These are questions no mortal can yet answer. Could life on earth be just part of a master plan for the universe? Are events described in "the prophecy" predestined or is man given choices through which he can alter his future?

I believe man is given opportunities and choices for a reason.

Fred Russell, vice-president of the *Nashville Banner*, once said: "the game we call Life got off to an unusual start. The Referee explained the rules; the rules got broken right off the bat; a penalty was inflicted. You may ask what was unusual about that? Well, it was the severity of the penalty—banishment forever from the Garden, and the guilty man would henceforth have to work for a living." Following that event, God intended for us to have some control over our destiny here on earth. He expects us to use our abilities and talents to become the best that we can be. The Bible tells us not to let the world squeeze us into its mold. (Roman 12:1-2) We may be just tenants on this planet, but we have an obligation while we are here—an obligation to ourselves and to our Creator. We are told of the physical signs (earthquakes, wars, floods, droughts, etc.) that precede the end of time on earth and that "such things must happen." Maybe we have no control over the destiny of planet Earth itself, but we must play the game to the best of our abilities until time runs out.

John Croyle, the founder of the Big Oak Boy's Ranch has often said, "A problem defined is 90% solved." An individual who understands *who he is* and *where he is going* is probably going to get there.

Although my life may represent only a tiny speck in this macrocosm, while climbing the mountain to become a facial surgeon, I have crossed the paths of some great men. Come with me and take a syllogistic look at real life situations from yesterday and today, and delve into some of the interpersonal relationships which I have been fortunate to develop with a few giants who were, and are, my teachers. Examine some adversities and hurdles I have had to challenge, with some yet to conquer. Look with me at some problems which must be resolved to insure America's continued existence and good health. View the world as I have seen it, from the shoulders of giants. Share with me decisions I made which helped me realize that I could and should do something meaningful. That is my destiny. It is my choice.

CHAPTER 2

A SEED IS PLANTED IN THE WIREGRASS

"Build me a son whose heart will be clear, whose goal will be high, a son who will master himself before he seeks to master other men, one who will reach into the future, yet never forget the past."

General Douglas MacArthur wrote those words to his son during the early days of World War II.

My roots were planted in an area of the Deep South called "The Wiregrass" by immigrants from Scotland and Ireland. O.E. McCollough and Gladys Wilson were born into large farming families of meager means in rural Alabama. You know the old tale about walking five miles to school each morning after doing one's chores. . . ., well, it was true in their lives.

During their early years of marriage they worked as share-croppers. My father plowed a mule until late afternoon and then frequently shot a wild rabbit for dinner. His wages each month totalled about $10.00.

Looking for a better way of life, he left the farm and asked an uncle to teach him how to become a plumber. Trading his plow for a wrench, he moved into a small town in southeastern Alabama.

When World War II started, as did most of his peers, he laid down his tools, took up a rifle and was off to fight the Japanese in the Aleutian Islands, near Alaska. My mother, then carrying me, waited patiently for his return.

I was brought into the world in Enterprise, Alabama on July 19, 1943. My father did not see me until I was a year old. During my early childhood, however, I did not lack guidance and attention. A positive self-esteem was cultivated early. An older uncle (Dudley Littleton) was my father-figure while my real father was away. He and Cleon, his wife, never had children of their own. I was fortunate that they became my godparents. During my first four years I spent more time with adults than with children. My parents had many adult friends who had no children, and I became part of their group.

In many respects, my childhood was short. Early in life I learned to think like an adult. Because of that, I have always felt comfortable around people who were older. I remember hearing my parents and their friends discuss job opportunities which passed them by because they were never able to get the education that they desired. Their choices were limited.

They wanted me to have a better chance. My parents planted the seeds early. They would often say: "Son, we want you to have the education that we never had. We will help you as much as we can. We want you to go as far as you can go, *even if you choose to be a doctor.* It may be necessary to mortgage everything we have, but we will see you through." They never came right out and said, "We want you to be a doctor." They were wise and knew how to work on me until it was my idea.

Someone once said,

> *"Discipline, like the bridle in the hand of a good rider, should exercise its influence without appearing to do so; should be ever active, both as a support and as a restraint, yet seem to lie easy in hand. It must always be ready to check or to pull up, as occasion may require; and only when the horse is a runaway should the action of the curb be perceptible."*[1]

Susan and I have tried this approach with our children, always em-

---

[1] *Treasury of Familiar Quotations,* p. 79.

phasizing the importance of high standards, education, and career planning, but allowing them to choose which fields they wish to pursue. We believe that Sted and Chanee must become his or her own person and do something that fits his or her individual make-up and personality. Too often, parents try to make children into clones of themselves. In doing so, they frequently drive wedges between the healthy parent-child relationship.

A Better Way

I saw my father work from early morning until late at night—repairing leaky faucets, stopped up toilets, and piecing steel pipe together when it was so cold that water had frozen to burst them. My mother worked as his bookkeeper and secretary. I didn't know people did anything but work, so, I worked too. Admittedly, like any normal child, I did not always want to, but my parents knew what they were doing by seeing that these work opportunities presented themselves.

From the time I was six, I was a peanut vendor, had newspaper routes, mowed lawns, and, as I got older, worked in the fields on farms, picking cotton, stacking peanuts, and doing numerous other jobs. When I became 16, I was allowed to work on construction jobs as a laborer.

This exposure to hard labor made me realize that a good education was the only answer to a better way of life. During the summer of 1960, prior to my graduation from high school, I was digging a ditch with a co-worker. He was 60 years old and had seven children. Each of us was earning a dollar and ten cents per hour. After several hours, we had dug the ditch to about six feet. As each shovel full of dirt was thrown out onto the bank being created beside the ditch, most of it would come down on us. Within a month I would be back in school, but he would be in another ditch somewhere else. At this time, he had no choice. I did. That is when I finally made the decision to get all of the education I could ("even if I choose to become a doctor").

My alternatives were clear. I could work hard for the rest of my life, or with the proper education, I could work smarter. Hard work, without the proper tools and knowledge, does not necessarily get the job done.

There is a story about the mechanic who was called to do a job because an expensive piece of equipment would not work. He took one minute to survey the situation, reached for a screwdriver and turned a screw one and a half turns. Immediately, the machine functioned properly. He was asked his fee for the job, to which he replied, "One hundred dollars." In amazement, the operator of the machine exclaimed, "One hundred dollars for a minute's work?!" "No", the mechanic replied, "for knowing which screw to turn and how far to turn it."

My dad has often said, "You can lose your home, your car and all your money, but no one can take away your education. As long as you have it, you have a chance to get all those material things back." I know my father had never read the works of Aristotle, who, when asked how much educated men were superior to those who were uneducated, answered, "as much as the living are to the dead."

In my mother's eyes, I could do no wrong. She made me believe that I was capable of accomplishing any goal I identified and was always there to catch me when I stumbled. Someone once said, "Because God could not be everywhere, He gave us mothers." Maybe my parents didn't have a great deal of formal education, but they sure had been blessed with common sense and knew about morals, ethics, and the value of an education. In one respect, however, they had the qualities of genius, which C. W. Ceram defined as "the ability to reduce the complicated to the simple."

My parents learned the value of education by the trial and error method, and wanted to see that I had a better chance than they had. They knew how to boost me up on their shoulders so that I could see what needed to be done.

Life is an evolutionary process. Each phase is a stepping stone onto the next. Harold V. Melchert advised us to, "Live life each day as you would climb a mountain. An occasional glance toward the summit keeps the goal in mind, . . . Climb slowly, steadily, enjoying each passing moment; and the view from the summit will serve as a fitting climax for the journey."[2]

The heights we achieve are determined by the goals we set.

Man can't hit a target he can't see. He can't climb a mountain he can't find. He can't control a destiny he can't perceive. My parents pointed me in the right direction and provided the propulsion for me to reach my target.

---

[2]*Motivational Quotes*, p. 54.

CHAPTER 3

FERTILE SOIL

"With a good heredity, nature deals you a fine hand at cards; and with a good environment, you learn to play the hand well."[1]

"Enterprise" is an international word which means, "being ready to undertake new or risky projects."[2] It was the name given to a space shuttle and a nuclear powered warship. It is also the name of my hometown.

I grew up in southeastern Alabama, in a small town founded upon a strong work ethic. Enterprise, Alabama, has established a tradition of excellence. That tradition is more than 100 years old. It shows no signs of being antiquated. Although some may consider tradition an intangible asset, it is as real as life itself. When it is alive it pulsates, particularly when it is built upon pride, dignity, and the willingness to accept any challenge with a total commitment to succeed. That desire to win and to achieve earned Enterprise and its people the reputation of a model American community. I was fortunate to have been part of the strong educational and athletic programs in Enterprise. The solid foundation I obtained in those programs allowed me to step further into a university football career which would open many doors

---

[1]Walter C. Alvarez, M.D., *Peter's Quotations.*
[2]*Webster's New World Dictionary,* p. 237.

for me and teach me innumerable lessons, particularly about dealing with people and conflicts. Later, I would have the opportunity to draw upon those experiences.

Make Something Happen

For those who have never had the opportunity to participate in the arena, there is an alternative. Like life itself, the game of football is a complicated interchange between people who perform, who teach, who watch, who simply talk about doing something, and who appear not to care about what happens. As with life, non-participants often try to be self-appointed "experts." Monday morning quarterbacks have 20/20 hindsight which they use to examine things more closely through "retrospectoscopes." They represent the "eye" of public opinion.

The football fan participates vicariously by watching others play. Although he might never put on the cleats, he represents one of the most essential elements of the game because he is a reflection of community involvement. Without a large contingency of demanding supporters, no tradition could survive very long. They provide the pulse of any sound program, spreading enthusiasm around the community.

It is when people stop talking that it is time to worry. A former Alabama governor, Big Jim Folsom, relished repeating an ancient axiom: "I don't care what people say as long as they say something and spell my name right."

What people say, however, is important. A good name is to be coveted. Like tradition, personal and professional reputations are not built overnight.

As I would soon discover, the higher one ascends the mountain toward his chosen destiny, the more often is he subjected to assaults by those who, because of envy, greed or jealousy, would attempt to tear him down by loose talk and malicious actions. Actually, a critic is an asset. If one has backbone, such a challenge from detractors generally adds force to his commitment and gives him added strength to overcome adversity.

Community success is no different. It has been said that, "all that is required for evil to prevail is that good men do nothing."

For this reason, good people must step forward and assume leadership roles knowing the risks they assume. Coaches and athletes recognize this fact. They do their parts on the field; they lay it all on the line. For the partnership to succeed, the community must do its share. People can be divided into three groups: those who do not know what happens; those who watch things happen; and those who make things happen.

Depending upon their levels of involvement, sports fans represent all three categories. The key is one's *level* of involvement. Supporting the dreams of young people can help make things happen for them and return dividends to the community.

Many fans know much less about the game than they would ever admit. Some don't know how much they don't know. People who should know better frequently overlook the human element of the game. Too often, we forget that those players on the field are still young men and women growing in mind, maturity and stature. Although everyone recognizes that human beings are far from being perfect, when a teenage boy suits up in his football gear, fans expect him and 10 others just like him to perform without mistakes.

Commitment is the Key

Any task that involves individual performance is fraught with the potential of error. Even those considered to be "experts" by their colleagues are unable to control every event around them. Since the Garden of Eden man has been imperfect. His destiny was altered when he chose to defy God's law. Man is a composite, a product of both genetics and environment. The actions of people around him affect his behavior and influence the outcome of many of his personal objectives, be it athletics, school, politics, or business. Regardless of how hard he may try, he will never be able to please everyone. People's opinions are generally biased, depending upon whether they agree or disagree with our own convictions. Those who make things happen expect to be subjected to criticism. Some things are beyond our control. When people criticize us, generally they do not understand WHY we choose to do the things we do. The person who sets his goals high will stumble along the way, but should keep in mind that, "In great attempts, it is glorious even to fail."[3]

---

[3]Anonymous, *Motivational Quotes* p. 73.

Football coaches and their players are expected to win, therefore fans allow them few mistakes. Their activities are closely examined by critics—fans and the media. Athletic mistakes are difficult to hide and poorly tolerated, especially in a community where winning is important.

What does all this have to do with tradition?

When the citizens of a community demand more from their coaches, teachers and players, the coaches, teachers, and players demand more from themselves. That's the cornerstone of tradition.

Millford Kelly was my high school English teacher. On several occasions, he returned my compositions with a grade of *C +*. I knew mine were better than those of classmates who got *A's*. When I confronted him about this, Mr. Kelly told me that as long as I gave him only 78 percent of my ability, he would give me 78 percent of the possible score. From that day forward, I set my standards higher, and the compositions improved. So did my scores!

Due to decades of intensive community involvement, Enterprise has enjoyed winning athletic programs documented by the records of its coaches: Russell Taylor, Herb Hawkins, Morris Higginbotham, Paul Terry and, currently, Bill Bacon. When the people of a community lose their interest in helping maintain a winning tradition, no program will remain at the top for very long.

Coach Vince Lombardi carved a place in history because of his commitment to winning. "Quality," he said, "is in direct proportion to the commitment to excellence." "Winning is not a sometime thing; it's an all-the-time thing." He continued, "You don't win once in a while, you don't do things right once in a while, you do them right all the time. Winning is a habit. Unfortunately, so is losing."[4]

A repeated thought becomes an action. A repeated action becomes a habit. Any tradition requires commitment and perpetual care so that being *in first place* continues to be THE way of life—a commitment to excellence. Unlike most habits, this one is difficult to acquire. It is even more difficult to maintain. Once one has sampled success, he is hooked. Nothing else ever tastes as good. Coach Paul Bryant often said, "Winning isn't everything, but it sure beats coming in second."

Winning is one habit no one wants to break.

---

[4]*Motivational Quotes,* p. 84.

Good Stock

How is the appetite of tradition fed? Tradition survives by invest-ing in young people. The grandstands at sporting events are often filled with former players. A player's love for competition and the de-sire to see his former athletic program prosper does not end the day he stops playing. A community must continue to feed its tradition with unwavering support. Many of the sons of former players carry on where fathers left off. More than likely, third generation sons will wear the same uniforms, the tradition passed along.

Loyal fans, good coaches, and community support are only part of the formula for preserving traditions. One of the most essential ele-ments in any project, athletics or otherwise, is the raw material used for the development of a final product, in this case the players. It stands to reason that the quality of the raw material usually deter-mines the quality of the product—quality in, quality out.

The southeastern area of Alabama is blessed with God-fearing, hard-working people. The pioneers literally dug its cities, roads, and fields from pine thickets, pulled up the roots of the trees with their mules, and worked the land with their hands. No one gave them any-thing but a chance to succeed. In the early days, boll weevils almost destroyed the economy, but the citizens didn't surrender in the face of adversity. They chose to fight back, not to be defeated by pests or hard times. They adapted, changing their crops from cotton to pea-nuts—a "new and risky project." When the cotton pest had nothing upon which to feed, he was no longer a problem. To their delight, they found the land was better suited for growing peanuts. The economy rebounded and the citizens prospered.

Adversity often turns out to be a blessing. In the end, the citizens of Enterprise erected a monument to the boll weevil, right smack in the middle of town, as a symbol of their toughness and commitment not to be defeated. It's not the Taj Mahal, but it is symbolic of pride and dignity—a victory over adversity. The monument's plaque reads: "December 11, 1919. In profound appreciation of the Boll-weevil and what it has done as the herald of prosperity. . ."

The *Book of Lists* calls the statue the most unusual in the world. It is the world's only glorification of an insect.

Like their forebearers, the young people reared in this region cer-tainly provide the raw materials necessary to develop any successful venture. They are of good stock.

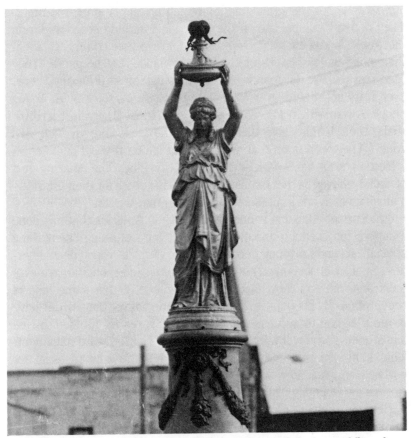

The Boll Weevil Monument, Enterprise, Alabama. It is the world's only glorification of a pest—a symbol of conquering adversity.

To Become a Hero

More importantly, however, Enterprise has made the commitment to excellence important to the young men who grow up there. The community has chosen to make them and their coaches heroes. The *American Heritage Dictionary* defines "hero" as one recognized for "feats of courage or nobility of purpose." Striving for excellence is "nobility of purpose."

It is difficult to place a value on the role personal recognition plays in bolstering one's self-esteem. There is no doubt, however, that it fulfills one of the basic needs of human existence. The players recognize whether the grandstands are full or empty on game night. They notice if people are on the sidelines watching practice during the week. Young ears anxiously listen for favorable comments about their potential as players or their performances in the game. They read newspapers or search to see their names in print anywhere, even if its just listed as one among 50 others on the roster. Young people swell with pride when people recognize them in a crowd, shake their hands, give them pats on the back and say "job well done." They feed upon recognition. That is one reward high school athletes get for hard work and personal sacrifice. The amazing part of it all, however, is that that is all they ask in return for their efforts— a small investment to preserve a tradition that works.

Enterprise, Alabama is one community in America that has done a superb job creating and nurturing that aura of being "something special" around its young people. They have made young people heroes. Smaller children see how any community responds to achievement and one day they hope to have a piece of that same kind of recognition. By choosing to keep the tradition alive, the citizens have paved the road to success and opened the gates for future athletes and students who will want to walk down the path toward fulfillment. This kind of community support provides the raw material for coaches and teachers who will ultimately develop young men and women into winning players and responsible citizens.

Being a "winner" must continue to be important to young people. In many communities around this country, many of the largest, fastest and strongest young men hang out at the soda shops in the afternoon rather than being at football or basketball practice. High school coaches depend upon community support in order to make athletics important to young people so that they want to participate.

From the Top

A "role model" has been defined as, "an individual that serves as a model . . . for another individual to emulate." Having the right role model is a key ingredient for a young person. He is the one who molds boys into young men. How does any community select one of the high school athlete's role model—his coach? Someone has to shoulder the responsibility to identify the right man and provide him with the physical plant needed to carry out his program. The school board of

Enterprise has seen to it that the people who run its educational and athletic programs are top-notch, well-qualified people. Someone once said, "The best executive is the one who has sense enough to pick good men to do what he wants done, and self-restraint enough to keep from meddling with them while they do it."[5]

Beginning years ago with R. L. Bates and Royce Snellgrove, then Oscar Zeanah, and now Thad Morgan and Coach Alfred Pevy, the community has been blessed with solid leaders who have a firm grip on today's activities and the foresight to plan for the future. These men and women chose to provide students with unequaled physical facilities and have seen to it that the athletic programs are run by coaches who know how to mold young men's futures.

Respect for people and property are the result of strong leadership and unwavering discipline, both of which have always existed among the school's officials and coaches.

Fans and parents do not always agree with every decision that school officials make. The important thing, however, is that we support their program and realize that these individuals were hired because *they* are the experts. Until an overall performance record indicates otherwise, no one can afford to tamper with success. If it ain't broke, don't fix it! Change is not necessarily synonomous with progress.

History teaches us that no leader reigns forever. The day comes when a coach's record may dictate a change, but that decision should not be based upon the outcome of a single game, or two, or even three. After our team has been beaten, it is human nature to question the leadership ability and judgement of any coach and transfer our frustrations to others. Like elevators, people, business and athletic programs go through the full cycle of ups and downs. The important thing is not to get stuck at the bottom.

Keep Your Head

After a losing game, even the most unsophisticated observer can identify specific situations when another strategy decision might have been better than one made at the time. After a loss, no coach's mind is idle. He second- guesses himself, exploring the other options

---

[5]*Motivational Quotes*, p. 5.

available and doing so in much more detail and with much more insight than those of us who were not there at the time the decision had to be made. He knows if he made the right decision and usually does not need for us to tell him so. He, above all others, knows if he is doing a good job. He expects to be replaced if he doesn't.

All who are placed in the position to make decisions expect to be questioned or criticized. Anyone who transends mediocrity will be challenged. Given the opportunity, his critics will attempt to pull him down. Rudyard Kipling in his poem "If" advises us how to deal with adversity when he writes "keep your head when others about you are losing theirs and blaming it on you, but make allowances for their doubting too. . ."

In the late 1960's, when the University of Alabama had two or three lackluster years, the so-called experts were calling for Coach Bryant's resignation. After that time, however, his team won several Southeastern Conference championships, a couple of national championships, and the 130 more games needed to reach the magic number of 323 making him the winningest *major* college coach of all time. In this case, many so-called experts were wrong again. Even a Monday morning quarterback would have called a wrong play if Coach Bryant had been forced to retire at that time. Public opinion must not make us deviate from what we know to be right and honorable.

A Part of Success

Lest we be too difficult on the Monday morning quarterback, we must remember that it is because observers feel that we know something about the game and understand some of its strategy that we feel obliged to express our own opinions. I can never remember questioning a decision made by a hockey coach, because I never cultivated an interest in the sport. I rarely understood WHAT was happening much less WHY it happened, what went wrong or what else could have been done.

When fans stop participating in the only way they know, and stop being Monday quarterbacks, athletic programs die from lack of interest.

Naturally, when our team wins, we share in the glory of the victory. We are quick to take some of the credit. We proudly proclaim, "That is MY team from MY hometown and I helped rear that kid who scored the winning touchdown or goal." We are proud to display OUR trophies, to be a part of success.

On the other hand, many of us tend to scatter when we are called upon to accept any part of failure. Although nothing about losing is considered good, lessons can be learned. Winning always seems better. It is human nature to make excuses when we lose and attempt to shift the blame elsewhere—to coaches, referees, the home field advantage, the weather, or to the turf. Like it or not, a final score is permanent. It is a piece of history. Nothing can erase it or alter it. Many times we can't even justify it. The best medicine is to swallow it and quickly hunt up another opportunity.

The Response to Failure

While playing football at Enterprise and at the University of Alabama, when we lost a game, we could hardly wait until the next week so that we could make things right again. Coach Bryant told us, after we lost, to watch for the following things: "First the crowd will be smaller outside the dressing room than it would have been had you won. Your parents and girlfriend may be out there. Your momma will hug you and say, 'We still love you.' Your daddy will shake your hand and say, 'That's okay son, we'll get them the next time,' but pay close attention to the differences in the quality of hugs and handshakes and listen for sincerity in their voices. Your girlfriend will kiss you politely, but there will be no passion in her embrace. She may hold your hand while you walk with her, but then again, she may not. Your folks will take you out to dinner and buy you a steak, but it won't taste very good. People who ordinarily look you up to say hello will find reasons to avoid you."

Coach was right. We felt uncomfortable with ourselves. We hated every minute of every day of the week after a loss. In general, the response to failure is negative. Life is just not as much fun because people don't like to associate with losers.

I seem to remember the details of every one of those games we lost. From the time I played varsity football in high school until I graduated from the University of Alabama, our teams lost only five (5) games. All the victories were more or less taken for granted because we *expected* to win every game we played. Winning had become a habit. The most satisfying wins were the ones following a loss from the previous week because we had made things "right" again. We simply did not know how to act when we lost. More importantly, not one of us wanted to get accustomed to it. Losing can become a habit, too—a habit that must not be tolerated.

The Test of Time

Although the emphasis was on winning, Coach Bryant taught us that even though you don't have to like losing, when it happens, you must maintain your dignity and demonstrate that you have class. That's self-control. When you've just been beaten, that's the time to make plans, not excuses. I can't ever remember hearing him make an excuse about losing, not to his players, to his coaches, or to the media. He always took the blame for losing and gave his players and assistant coaches the credit for winning. One must have a strong ego to shoulder such responsibility. He was a role model for all Americans. Role models are important in times of stress and dismay. It is during periods of confusion and disharmony that we turn to principles that have endured the test of time.

Augustus Caesar recognized the basis of his heritage and Rome's strength. He warned that even a great civilization requires constant attention in order to perpetuate itself. In a statement to the younger generation of his Empire he advised, "Young men, hear an old man to whom old men hearkened when he was young."[6] Unfortunately, the young people of Rome neither heard nor took heed. The rest is history.

As parents, teachers and civic leaders, it is our duty to pass along a tradition that works to our sons and daughters. Then, it is their responsibility to see that the chain remains unbroken.

The community of Enterprise is rich in its tradition and strong in its heritage. Its principles have stood the test of time. Many of its citizens may not fully appreciate what a strong foundation their forebears established. For many years to come, pride, honor, dignity, and the desire to excel will continue to echo in the halls of its schools and churches and live within the hearts and minds of all those who have had the good fortune to be touched by it.

The community should never lose its obsession for excellence. It

---

[6]*Bartlett's Quotations.*

must never withdraw its full support from the people it has entrusted to carry on the tradition. It must continue to make its educators, coaches, and players heroes, but, most of all, must never let its passion for excellence slip.

Portrait of a Football Player

Participation in athletics can be compared to living the game of life. The way we play it usually determines its ultimate outcome—a destiny of choice. The lessons learned through athletics will serve one well throughout the rest of his life. A day never passes that I don't use some lesson about teamwork or self-sacrifice that I learned from football, basketball or baseball. Those who are associated with athletics are probably better citizens because of it, and better prepared for the test of life.

In America, the athlete always has been and always will be "something special." What makes him so special? Several years ago, Fred Russell sent me a clipping from the school newspaper at Red Bank School in Chattanooga. With some literary license, I will attempt to paint the portrait of a football player.

"Sandwiched between the innocence of boyhood and the dignity of man, we find a sturdy young creature called a football player. Hustle is his middle name—trying is his game.

Football players come in assorted weights, heights, jersey colors and numbers; but all have the same goal—to play every second of every game to the best of their abilities for themselves and their school.

On game day football players are found everywhere—underneath, on top of, running around, jumping over, passing by, twisting from, or driving through the opposing team. Throughout the rest of the week they practice, study, dream and scheme.

Their own teammates tease them, officials penalize them, fellow students cheer them, kid brothers idolize them, coaches and fans criticize them, girls adore them, fathers brag about them, and mothers worry about them.

A football player is courage in cleats, hope in a helmet, pride in pads, and exemplifies the very best of America's young manhood.

His coaches try to make him believe he can perform like an All-American, but more often than not, he falls far short of these expectations.

The same football player may appear to be a totally different individual, depending upon who is describing him. To an opponent coach, he may be said to have: the speed of a deer, the strength of an ox, the size of an elephant, the cunning of a fox, the agility of a dancer, the quickness of a cat, and the ability of Joe Namath, Lee Roy Jordan, Cornelius Bennett, and Bo Jackson combined; however, when his own coach describes him to the press before the game, he has the stability of potato soup, the fleetness of a snail, the mentality of a mule, and is being held together by adhesive tape, bandaids, bailing wire and sponge rubber. He will probably come to the stadium on crutches and has about as much chance of playing well as would his own grandfather.

To an alumnus, who played "back when," today's football player is someone who will never kick as well, run as fast, block as viciously, tackle as hard, fight as ferociously, give as little ground, score as many points, or generate nearly as much school spirit as did the particular players of his own yesteryear.

In stadiums all around America, people gather to watch him and his teammates determine the outcome of the game fans hope to boast about during the coming week.

Whether we are a parent, an alumnus, a coach or fan—he is our personal representative on the field—our symbol of fair play and hard work. He may not be an All-American, but he is an example of the American way. He will not be judged for his race, religion, social standings, or finances (you see, football uniforms have no pockets). He is judged by his performance—the democratic yardstick of how well he blocks, tackles, and sacrifices individual glory for the overall success of his team.

The football player is a hardworking, untiring, determined young man doing the very best he can for his school and asking very little in return. So the next time we leave a stadium disgusted and feeling upset that our team has lost, if we were to meet him face to face, with tears of disappointment in his eyes, he can make us feel almighty ashamed with just two sincerely spoken words—"We tried."

Although disappointed and temporarily beaten, he won't give up—that's not his style. On Monday, we can find him at practice, working to get ready to come back the following week and "try again."

That's where we need to be, too. We need to show him that we're still behind him. That's what preserves successful programs, strong traditions and self-esteem.

The people of Enterprise, Alabama never gave up on their young people. They have always been there when needed. I am proud to be a product of the Enterprise tradition. That heritage and those roots are important to me. The years I spent there provided the foundation upon which I have established my goals and my principles.

Our roots allow us to branch out from a solid foundation. We build upon the past and look toward the future, gazing into the face of our own destiny.

Looking Forward

Young people looking for direction can turn to Winston Churchill. In a challenge to us all, he advised,

> *"Come on now all you young men all over the world. . .*
> *Don't be content with things as they are. . . Enter into your*
> *inheritance, accept your responsibilities. . . Don't take no*
> *for an answer, never submit to failure. Do not be fobbed off*
> *with mere personal success or acceptance. You (will) make*
> *all kinds of mistakes; but as long as you are generous and*

true, and also fierce, you cannot hurt the world or even se-
riously distress her. . . she is made to be wooed and won by
youth."[7]

Fortunately, around the United States, there are many communities like Enterprise, who are ready "to undertake new and risky projects." That's what makes this country envied. Unfortunately, however, in some communities, adults seem to get all wrapped up in their own activities and in climbing the social ladder, and fail to recognize that the best investment one can make in his community is to support those programs which help its young people mature into responsible citizens.

Enterprise is one example of the American way, a community that has done it the right way, by investing in its youth. By putting that little "extra" into the future of its youth, the tradition is insured.

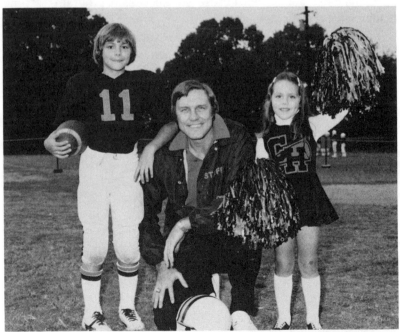

"Coach" Gaylon McCollough with Sted and Chanee during their younger
days with the Cahaba Heights Black Knights.

---

[7]Bartlett, *While England Slept* p. 920.

PART II

A LOOK AT MANHOOD

CHAPTER 4

THE RING

"Once to every man . . . comes the moment to decide. . ."[1]

In every young man's life, the moment comes when he must decide upon a career, a choice of destiny. That's when he becomes an adult. Generally, this is done in a methodical manner with consultation and without outside pressures. For the graduating high school athlete who is being recruited to participate in intercollegiate athletes, the process can be mind boggling, especially, if no one in his family attended college.

At the age of 17, I found myself having to make a decision that would determine my life's work. Because I had the good fortune to play on a state championship high school football team and received All-State honors, my parents and I were contacted by a number of colleges and universities offering four year athletic scholarships. The scholarship would provide the necessary amenities and allow me to obtain a college education while participating in its athletic program.

Today, there is much controversy over the student-athlete not completing his college curriculum or getting his degree. No one can deny that each one of them should take advantage of the educational opportunity. If, however, it were not for the chance to go to college on an athletic scholarship, some underprivileged young men and

---

[1] J. R. Lowell, "The Present Crisis," *The Pocket Book of Quotations* p. 60.

women might never even see a college campus, meet a Ph.D., or see that a better way of life is theirs for the taking. There is no excuse for lack of effort, but let us not become so idealistic in our thinking that we ignore the good that can come from the college experience. There may be a place for a separate set of standards, even if it means affiliation with a trade school.

What is wrong, however, is for the student-athlete to go to college with his hand out and expect to be given anything but an opportunity.

In 1985, the College Football Association (CFA) initiated a series of 30-second testimonials during their televised games to offset some of the negative publicity surrounding academics in intercollegiate sports.

The CFA asked each of its 80 members to submit a name of a former player who needed an athletic scholarship in order to attend college. Specifically, it wanted names of those who had used that experience as a stepping stone into the business and professional world.

The University of Alabama submitted my name for consideration. I was honored to be one of 16 men chosen from across America to do the spots which were aired during half-time of the weekly college games. I believe the campaign was effective. I only hope the young student-athletes grasped the message we were sending.

Athletics can provide an opportunity to obtain an education which allows one to control his own destiny. My scholarship was a crucial first step into a better way of life. I am grateful to have had the opportunity to share my feelings with the young people of America.

Choices

Because of the scholarship offer, it appeared that a college education was going to be available without my father having to mortgage our home. After discussions with several universities (Clemson, Florida State, Auburn, Georgia Tech, and Alabama), the choice was narrowed to two: Georgia Tech and the University of Alabama.

Throughout high school, I had been an Auburn fan, having attended band camp there for two consecutive summers. My idols were Zeke Smith, now a member of the Alabama Sports Hall of Fame and Ed Dyas, who became a doctor and a member of the selection committee for the Hall of Fame. Many of my friends and teammates were planning to attend Auburn. The campus was close to home, and, therefore provided an element of convenience.

During my junior year in high school, I had been one of the representatives from Enterprise to the State of Alabama's Boy's State Convention at the University of Alabama. I was comfortable with the campus, impressed with its academic standards, and familiar with its strong football tradition. I also liked the sound of *"The* University of Alabama."

Florida State was recruiting me as a quarterback (so it said) and had offered to extend my scholarship through medical school at the University of Florida. (I often wonder if that could have been possible). I had been a quarterback in high school until our new coach (Morris Higginbotham) came to town and eliminated the T-formation offense. According to the Florida State recruiter during the spring game before Coach Higginbotham came, he had seen some potential as a college quarterback. I was tall, strong, and had a good passing arm for their pro-type passing offense. Who wouldn't rather play quarterback than center? I was afraid that the Florida State recruiter was using the "promise them anything" tactic.

Medicine vs. Architecture

During those days, I had a friend who was studying architecture at Georgia Tech on a football scholarship and was a member of the Tech team. Ed Chancey had been an All-American young man in Enterprise and emerged as a high school role model for many of us a few years younger. Needless to say, the academic reputation of Georgia Tech, the encouragement from Ed, and my own interest in architecture made that option very appealing.

The University of Alabama's national academic status, its reputation and commitment to excellence, the fact that Coach Bryant was there to re-establish its football supremacy, and the University's recognized pre-med program, I reasoned, could serve as a stepping-stone into Alabama's medical school in Birmingham. These factors made Alabama a very attractive choice.

My career decision was soon narrowed to architecture at Georgia Tech or medicine at the University of Alabama. It was a choice that would determine my life's work. My destiny was hanging in the balance.

As signing day approached, I vacillated between the two schools, realizing that either decision could offer me an outstanding career opportunity. During this time, my parents would only ask questions to make me think. They wanted the final decision to be my own.

My father had been involved in the construction business for most of his life and I had worked several summers on construction jobs. I knew something about the building industry. I had always enjoyed drawing and creating models of buildings and bridges with match sticks or erector sets. I knew nothing about medicine except that when I got sick, I went to the doctor and usually got a shot. After weeks of deliberation and many conversations with the Tech recruiter, Coach Jim Luck (now an assistant athletic director), I had decided that Georgia Tech and architecture was the way to go. In the back of my mind, however, I could still hear my dads words, ". . . even if you choose to be a doctor."

To Be a Champion?

Bob Ford was the coach from Alabama assigned to recruit me. One evening, while sitting at the breakfast table in our kitchen, I told Coach Ford that I thought I should go on over to Georgia Tech. He got very quiet and said, "Gaylon, I'm sure you can be happy there. If you go to Tech, you'll get a good education and win a lot of games and have a great college experience." Then, he reached over to his right ring finger and pulled off a magnificent gold ring with a diamond in its center. He handed it to me. "Do you know what this is?" he asked. I looked more closely and read the inscription on the ring. "SOUTHWEST CONFERENCE, TEXAS A&M, 1956." He looked me straight in the eye and asked, "Would you like to wear one like this someday?" He knew what I would answer and he continued; "If you come to Alabama, I can *guarantee* you that before you leave there you will play on a *national* championship team and own a championship ring." That is all it took. I chose the opportunity to once again be a champion.

It looked as though architecture would yield to medicine. Little did I know the two would come together for me in a field of medicine that I didn't even know existed at the time—facial plastic surgery.

I had already played on a state high school championship team.

Once you have been a champion, nothing less is satisfactory. I had been convinced that at Alabama, under the greatest coach who ever lived, I could once again play on a championship team.

My freshman year (1961), Alabama won the National Championship. My sophomore year a 7-6 loss to Georgia Tech (ironically enough) was all that kept us from repeating that championship. In 1964, my senior year, the dream would be realized. Bob Ford's "guarantee," the championship ring, and the pre-med college degree all would be a reality; but not without some difficult times.

Coach Bryant often said, "the price of victory is high, but so are the rewards." At that time, I did not realize how high the price was to be. Success was to be achieved through planning, organization, hard work, taking some lumps, assessing what had been done, adaptation and more hard work.

John Ruskin once wrote, "No great intellectual thing was ever done by great effort; a great thing can only get done by a great man, and he does it without effort."[2]

I'm not sure about "great intellectual" things, but I have learned that most of the great men who accomplished their personal goals did so with intelligence *and* a great deal of effort.

---

[2]George Seldes, "Pre-Raphaelitism," *The Great Thoughts* p. 360.

CHAPTER 5

THE CRIMSON JERSEY

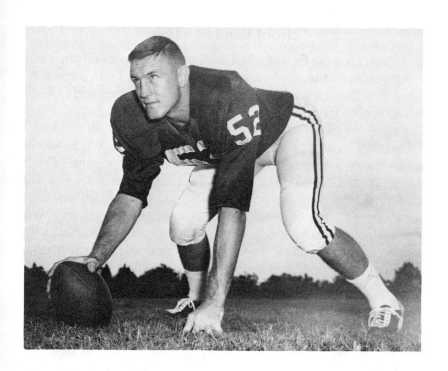

The trip from Enterprise to Tuscaloosa was only 200 miles, but on that day in August of 1961, it seemed as if it were 2,000. At age 17, the reality of leaving home hadn't really occurred to me, but as we drove into the parking lot at the athletic dormitory on the campus of The University of Alabama, the look on my mother's face told the entire story. She knew, better than I, that I was about to step into an entirely different world, beyond the security of family and hometown. Fortunately, I was carrying with me a solid foundation shored up by all those people who had helped me get to that point in my life.

Going away to college is a new beginning. Young Boozer, a Tuscaloosa businessman, said that his mother gave him good advice when he left Dothan to attend the University of Alabama. She told him, "you can pick your friends, but not your relatives. Work hard, tell the truth and associate with people who are smarter than you are."

It must have worked. He has done well.

School Comes First

My next home, in the old athletic dormitory (Friedman Hall), was a single room for two. As I walked through the door, I was surprised to see that the face across the room was the same one I had looked into across the line of scrimmage during the Alabama high school all-star game one month previously. There he stood, 6'1" tall, weighing 235 pounds, crew cut, arms like a weightlifter. I gulped. Was he waiting for me to get even for the outcome of the all-star game? Dan Kearley of Talladega had been an offensive tackle on the North squad. I had been a defensive linebacker on the South squad which won the game. We had been adversaries. Things were different now. We would become roommates, teammates, and friends. Isn't it strange how circumstances can change the way people look upon each other? Opponents became teammates; adversaries friends—the secret to existence in a nutshell.

After Dan and I got settled in our quarters, we had our first meeting with the man who was responsible for our being there. When Coach Bryant walked in, you could have heard a pin drop. He had "presence." There was an air of reverence throughout the room— his reputation had preceded him. A frightened, naive group of freshmen had heard the stories about those first years at Alabama and Texas A&M (the pit on the practice field, the "gut checks" and the No. 12 boots, especially the one he wore on his right foot).

It was somewhat eerie to know that this man held the reins to each of our athletic careers and my college education. He spoke with authority and purpose. "The first thing each one of you will do tonight is write home to your parents," he said. "Keep in touch with them and tell them you love them." Coach Bryant had a thing about family.

He made it clear that we were there to accomplish several goals, ours and his. "School comes first", he said, "because unless you make your grades, you won't be eligible to play; no matter how talented you are. You're a student first, then a football player." He felt strongly that an education was important to life after football. On that point, he and my father were in perfect agreement. Later, I discovered there were many other similarities.

In those days, more than 90 percent of his players earned their college degrees. He allowed them to come back and work with the athletic department while working toward their college degrees even though they had played out their eligibility. Everyone had the opportunity to complete academic requirements.

The Other Team

It didn't take long for us to get indoctrinated into college football. Freshmen could not participate in varsity athletics in those days, at least not in the games. Right away, however, we found ourselves being "the other team" during practice. Within a week, we were scrimmaging against the group that was to become the 1961 national championship team.

Each day I lined up opposite Charlie Pell, the former University of Florida coach. He has always been a fierce competitor. He hates losing. I saw this trait in him early as we fought it out each day at practice.

Charlie Pell was an outstanding football player and a good football coach. He had also climbed to the top quickly. Maybe his sudden success and passion to win contributed to his fall from grace. He lost his job at Florida following the NCAA's punitive sanctions, and Florida was no doubt guilty of the cited recruiting violations. Both of these factors made him vulnerable.

He has been critical of the NCAA, not because of what they did to him, but because they allow similar violations to occur at other institutions. The NCAA seems to turn their heads on the activities of some of their "sacred cows". That's what Charlie calls those who seem to be immune from the NCAA's wrath. He knows who the other violators are, but dislikes the NCAA so much that he refuses to help them "can" anyone else, even an adversary. Recently, Charlie has gone to work with a teammate and mutual friend, Curtis Crenshaw, who is the owner of Southcoast, a successful shopping center development corporation.

Charlie Pell is a survivor, I battled him almost every day for an entire season. When he gets it all together, he will rebound. That 1961 Alabama team went undefeated both in practice and during their regular schedule. The freshmen quickly learned what was to be expected from everyone who put on the crimson jersey, a symbol of Alabama's football tradition.

Our New Quarterback

All but one of our freshmen squad had reported to the University on time. About four days later, however, during practice, I looked over to the sidelines and saw a sporty looking young man standing there wearing a sport coat, tie, and a hat with a little feather sticking up on one side. He also had a toothpick in the corner of his mouth.

"Who is that character?" I asked one of the student assistant coaches. "Your new quarterback," he said. I chuckled and said, "He will last about two days." When I saw him walk over to the tower and climb up there with Coach Bryant, I knew he must be an extraordinary talent, because nobody, but nobody, went up on that tower with "the man."

Joe Namath was late in reporting because he had originally planned to play at the University of Maryland. Fortunately for Alabama he decided to come south instead.

A few days later Namath was directing our freshman team, using the Alabama offense against the 1961 varsity team, and doing it like a veteran. The toothpick did go after a few days, but the quarterback remained. He became a legend in his own right.

Our First College Game

On a hot, humid September afternoon, we went over to Starkville, Mississippi to play the Mississippi State freshman team. We only took about 20 players because Alabama had recruited a very small freshman class. In the average college game today, approximately 60 players participate in a game. This is the era of specialization in football, too. Players are offensive or defensive specialists, kicking specialists, short yardage specialists, etc. The era of playing both ways (offense *and* defense) is history.

In Starkville that afternoon, the temperature was in the high 90's and most of us played both offense and defense. Mississippi State had a good team and played us to the wire. Late in the fourth quarter, I thought I would drop from exhaustion. Clem Gryska, the freshman coach, took me out for a rest, three plays. Our offense stalled and we didn't make the first down, so he turned to me and said, "Gaylon, go back in there and snap the ball for the punt." I ran back onto the field.

The score was something like 20-14, so that if Mississippi State should score a touchdown and an extra point, they would beat us. We had the ball in our territory with just three or four minutes left in the game. The obvious strategy would be to punt the ball deep into Mississippi State territory and try to hold them until the clock ran out— obvious to everyone except Namath.

As I stepped into the huddle, Joe was calling *a pass play*. I thought, "He must not know it is fourth down." "Joe," I interrupted, "it is fourth down and I was sent in to snap for the punt." He said, "We can't punt if we are going to win this game. We have got to make a first down." I looked to the sideline and held up my hands to indicate that I had delivered the message.

Joe took the snap from me, stepped back three steps and drilled a perfect pass to our receiver for the first down. We ran out the clock and won the game. He knew how worn out we all were, and probably felt that if we punted, we could not cover the punt effectively. Mississippi State just might return it for a touchdown, or at least get a good return and put it in a position to score. After running to cover the punt, we would certainly be even more exhausted and would not be able to play adequate pass defense against the fresher Mississippi

State offense. They had played about 60 players throughout the game. Looking back, I am sure Joe knew exactly what he was doing. From that day on, I never questioned Joe's play calling. He recognized our limitations and his abilities. His choice was well founded—based upon knowledge, skills, courage and the confidence that if we made the first down, we were in control of our own destiny. He was and is a football genius.

The Cardiac Kids

My first game as an Alabama player had been won the old-fashioned way, with blood, sweat, and preparation. It set the stage for what was to follow during the next four years. Our group was later to be labeled "The Cardiac Kids" because we won so many close games in the waning minutes. When we stepped on the field in Starkville wearing those crimson jerseys, we knew we represented the Alabama tradition, and that we were going to be entrusted to carry it on.

Wrestling Class

During the "off season" we stayed in shape through an intensive physical fitness program. "Wrestling Class" as it was then called, was held three days each week in a small, gloomy gymnasium above the old coaches' and athletic offices on University Boulevard. Sometimes things got pretty testy during those work-outs. There was a tiny door which led out to the roof for those whose stomachs got upset causing them to throw-up. Wrestling partners were usually assigned by positions, i.e., quarterbacks wrestled quarterbacks, tackles wrestled tackles, and centers wrestled centers. My wrestling partner was none other than the concensus All-American (and later All-Pro with the Dallas Cowboys) Lee Roy Jordan. That was not by choice.

I could never quite decide if the coaching staff was trying to get me to quit or teaming me up with Lee Roy to keep him from getting hurt. Fortunately both of us survived, escaping without injury. During those sessions, I learned what the word "tough" really means. I believe the toughness learned during the off-season programs allowed us to win a couple of games at the wire during the championship season.

Winning Isn't Everything

Winning was the only way at Alabama. There was a plaque hanging behind Coach Bryant's desk in his office which stated, "Winning isn't everything, but it sure beats being second." Life wasn't much fun around Alabama after losing. Even as freshmen we already knew that much. We were afraid of what might happen to us if we came back to Tuscaloosa as losers. Not only the coaches, but the varsity players would make life miserable for us.

Coach Bryant was a great motivator and psychologist. He made us believe that nothing seems right when you lose. We looked for the difference and (guess what) it was there when we lost. We could hardly wait for next Saturday to make things right again.

During my entire career at Alabama, we never lost two games in a row. One loss, however, produced an indelible mark in my memory.

"Time Just Ran Out"

During my sophomore year, we were rated *No. 1* in the country by both major national polls going into our eighth game against Georgia Tech. The dream of owning a national championship ring was close to becoming a reality. We had an open date prior to that game, which allowed us additional time to prepare for a very good Tech team. Our 1962 Alabama team was also fortunate to have two quarterbacks who were great athletes, Joe Namath, a great passer, and Jack Hurlbut, a strong runner. The coaching staff came up with a new offensive scheme which, on paper, seemed unbeatable. The choice was made to change from the plan which allowed us to win eight consecutive games. With this new formation, we would have both of our quarterbacks in the game at the same time. Hurlbut would be in the usual position, behind the center; Namath would replace the fullback in a "shotgun" formation. Depending upon the situation we had the option either to snap the ball to Hurlbut in the usual fashion, to put Hurlbut "in motion," or to snap the ball through his legs to Namath and run plays from the "shotgun." We called the new offense "red, white, and blue," each color describing variations in the alignment of our backfield.

Quickly, one can see that the Tech defense should be caught off guard and have a great deal of difficulty in adjusting to this offensive

scheme. At least that is what should have happened. On the first play
of the game we lined up in our new formation.

Hurlbut went in motion and the Tech defensive captain called out
"blue . . . blue" and then made some adjustments. (That is exactly
what we had named that particular variation of our new offense).
They stopped the play for no gain. "Just a coincidence," I thought. On
the next play, we lined up and I snapped the ball through Hurlbut's
legs, back to Namath in the "shotgun" position. The Tech linebacker
called out "red . . . red" and they quickly adjusted (red formation
was the correct term for that offensive variation). The rest of the
first half went about as well. Georgia Tech had obviously prepared for
us. They stopped us cold during the first half. Our *unbeatable* new
offense fizzled. At halftime, Coach Bryant changed everything: he
adapted to the situation. He completely discarded the "red, white,
and blue" offense and drew on the blackboard of our dressing room
about a half dozen running plays and passes which we had used in
other games to get us to an 8-0 record and our No. 1 rating. We had
not practiced running some of these plays, however, for two weeks.
But we had to do something different. His ability to change course at
the right time was one of the secrets to his success.

During the second half, our team did better. We rallied from a 7-
0 deficit to score a touchdown late in the fourth quarter. Before attempting the extra point "time-out" was called. With about three or
four minutes left in the game, the decision was made by the coaching
staff to go for two points instead of kicking the one point extra point
play. If successful, we would go ahead by a score of 8-7 and Coach
Bryant felt our defense could hold Tech and run out the clock. The
strategy was sound. Hurlbut was a strong running quarterback and
Namath had been banged up during the game. So, Hurlbut was chosen to run a roll-out, or sweep play, around the right end. At the goal
line, a tremendous collision occurred with a Tech defender and the
official ruled that Hurlbut did not get into the end zone—but it was
not yet over.

With the score now Georgia Tech 7, Alabama 6, we kicked off and,
as predicted, held the Tech offense. Lee Roy Jordan, our great linebacker, helped cause a fumble at midfield and our offense went back
into the game to win it. After several successful plays, the ball was
resting inside Georgia Tech's 10 yard line. On third down, time was
called and a summit conference was held on the Alabama sideline. We

had an outstanding field goal kicker, Tim Davis (now an Ob-Gyn doctor in Birmingham), so, the question was to either kick the (winning)
field-goal on third down or run one more play and kick it on the fourth
down.

Coach Bryant told our quarterback to run a pass play and look for
Bill Battle, the former head coach at Tennessee, in the end zone. If
he was open, throw to him for the touchdown. If there was any Tech
player close to him, throw the ball over his head for an incomplete
pass and we would kick the (winning) field goal on fourth down.

When the play developed, Battle was covered, so Hurlbut threw
the ball high over his head, as directed. Bill Battle was a great athlete
and a fierce competitor. He jumped as high as he could trying to catch
the ball, only to reach it with part of one hand. The ball began to fall
to the ground like a wounded quail. As it did, however, it landed in the
outstretched hands of one of the Tech pass defenders. INTERCEP-
TION!!! Tech's ball on the 20 yard line.

It was just not meant for us to win on that day. As Georgia Tech
celebrated and ran off the remaining seconds on the clock, all our
players, coaches, and staff saw the national championship slip
through our grasps. The dream of winning the ring would have to
wait.

With his head held high and his back straight, Coach Bryant walked
to the center of the field and congratulated Coach Bobby Dodd. He
then went to the Georgia Tech dressing room and congratulated their
players. Then he walked over to our dismal dressing room and led us
in prayer (as he often did). His words that day, however, made a lasting impression on me. He said, "Dear Lord, please let these young
men forgive me. If I had stayed at home, they could have won."

The feeling in that dressing room in Atlanta that afternoon, following those words, turned from one of despair and self-pity to one of
pride and respect. Coach Bryant did not lose the game, we did. He
did not miss a tackle, fail to make a block, or drop a pass. We did all
of those things, but he accepted the blame for the defeat. Not one
excuse did he make nor did he criticize the officials, the Tech student
body (who had made standing on the sidelines dangerous that day),
nor any assistant coach or any of his players.

That was a special opportunity to see the character of this giant
of a man. Although he was not totally responsible for the outcome of
the game, he was "the boss" and accepted full responsibility for

everyone's actions when things went awry. On the other hand, he was quick to give all the credit to others when things went well. More on that theme later.

After Coach Bryant had concluded his remarks about the Georgia Tech game, he said, "this one is now history. You can walk out of this dressing room with pride and hold your heads up high. You men are not losers. You were not beaten today. *Time just ran out on you.*" That's the first time I had ever heard those words. "Next week", he said, "we play Auburn in Birmingham. You have a choice to feel sorry for yourselves and get beat, or you will have a full sixty minutes to continue what you started here today in the fourth quarter of this game. Now, let's put this one behind us and get ready for next week."

Picking Up the Pieces

It was hard to pick up the shattered dreams of a national championship, but life goes on and we did have a chance to prove something to ourselves and to our coach. Rudyard Kipling in "IF" states if you can "lose, and start all over at the beginning and never breathe a word about your loss. . . then, you'll be a man. . ."
The next week in Birmingham, we beat Auburn by a score of 38-0 and accepted an Orange Bowl bid to play Oklahoma, who had taken over our No. 1 rating, on New Year's Day. We won that game 17-0.

The 1962 Alabama team finished the season with a record of 10 wins and one loss (7-6). More than the record and a trip to Miami, however, I learned a lesson during a moment of despair in that dressing room in Atlanta that proved to be more valuable than another national championship ring. Defeat is a state of mind. Like elevators, champions can work their way right back up to the top after a big letdown. It is a matter of choice. I was later going to get a chance to prove to myself (off the field) that no condition is ever permanent, good or bad.

"Destiny . . . is a thing to be achieved."[1]

---

[1]William Jennings Bryan

CHAPTER 6

A YEAR OF BEING TESTED

With the graduation of several outstanding seniors and an injury to Joe Namath leaving the 1963 Alabama team with less experience and talent, we struggled through the season and ended with a 9-2 record. Our two losses were to Florida (10-6) and to Auburn (10-8), however, several of our victories were that close, too (Mississippi State 20-19 and the University of Mississippi, in the Sugar Bowl, 12-7).

The coaching staff was presented with a challenge: trying to come up with a winning combination in the starting lineup and making many of us play beyond our abilities. This created some extremely stressful situations, both mentally and physically. We were all "tested" to see how important football was to us and which ones would break under pressure. During that year, we had several "gut checks" on the practice field, which resulted in a number of players giving up football. Certainly each and everyone of us seriously considered quitting from time to time; however, Coach Bryant was a masterful motivator and psychologist. He knew human nature and knew how to identify winners.

A Rededication

Following a struggle to win a game from Vanderbilt University, he called an early morning meeting which was designed to "introduce" the old hard-nosed brand of football to those of us who had not been at Alabama when he came back from Texas A&M in 1958. We had heard the stories about how difficult things had been on a regular basis in those days and were concerned about what surely was to follow in the days ahead.

During that early morning meeting, "examples" were made of several players and one assistant coach as to what was to be unacceptable from that moment forward. Coach Bryant demonstrated the "proper" method of tackling on Charlie Pell, now an assistant coach, who had been late for the meeting—something no one dared to do. I was sitting in the front row and was afraid that at any minute I might be singled out for a demonstration.

Following that "rededication" gathering, five players went back to the football dormitory, packed their belongings and left for home. They chose to give up football. The rest of us waited to see what was going to transpire later that day during practice. That day must have been one of the longest of my life. I prayed that God would give me the strength once again to endure what might follow.

A "Gut-Check"

My memory went back a year to a hot April afternoon in 1962. It had been my first experience with one of Coach Bryant's "gut checks."

Spring training was always a time to get down to the nitty-gritty—that's when Coach Bryant separated the men from the boys. There was always at least one "gut check" during spring training but no one knew when it would occur.

The thermometer on the little branch bank across the street from the practice field read 102°. I often wondered if it had been placed there at the recommendation of the coaching staff to remind us just how hot it really was. It was a perfect setting to test commitment. Because most of us anticipated that this would be the day, before practice the dressing room was quiet. Each player was searching his soul like the soldier preparing for battle—making peace with himself and his Maker. As I pulled the practice jersey over my head, I said a little prayer during that brief moment of solitude when no one could see my face. I prayed for strength to endure whatever lay ahead.

I jogged onto the practice field (no one ever walked once he stepped foot on the field) wondering if I would be sent in (and home) before practice was over that day. After about an hour of "warm up drills" (the temperature was 102°) Coach Bryant blew the whistle for the scrimmage to begin.

The offense was given the ball on its own 20 yard line. We would have four downs to make a first down. No passes or punts were allowed. If the first down was made, the offense would have the opportunity to make another and another until a touchdown was scored. Following the score, the ball would be brought back to its original point, 80 yards away from the goal line. The entire process was repeated, over and over again. Such repetition was designed to instill confidence in an individual's (and a team's) ability to perform with precision and consistency in the face of fatigue.

So much for the "rewards" of such a scrimmage. What about the other side of the picture? If the defense stopped the offense from scoring or from making a first down, the offensive team would go over to the sidelines and run forty yard sprints while the defense rested and were congratulated by the coaching staff. When the sprints were completed, the offensive team would once again get the ball 80 yards from the goal line, and have the opportunity to mount a drive.

After the second set of sprints, I thought to myself, "I must rest. I don't think I can run another step." A little voice inside me said, "Keep going. You must do it." Looking back at that moment, I now know that practice was not yet half over.

My entire football career was riding on surviving the next two hours. Several times during that practice, I wanted to quit, but something drove me onward. Was it destiny? I shudder to think how different my life might have been had I chosen to give up.

Athletes often talk about getting their "second wind". Runners call it "going through the wall". At the point when the body says, "I can't," if the mind insists, eventually, the body responds by releasing a type of hormone called endorphins. They are natural narcotics produced by the body which ease pain and give a sense of well-being. Unless one has been pushed to the critical point, he never experiences the "natural high" which comes from "going through the wall". Once the barrier has been broken, the athlete then tests himself to see how much farther he can go. Knowing that this reserve is there tends to reduce the anxiety of fatigue. It is a frightful thing, however, the first time one experiences it.

I don't believe Coach Bryant knew about endorphins but he knew about pushing us until we either broke or until we got our "second wind." He called it a "gut-check." On that hot, muggy April afternoon, each player eventually got his "second wind", then the second part of the test began.

Our offensive team had driven the ball down the field to the one yard line. It was fourth down and goal to go. Coach Bryant was up in his observation tower watching every movement on the field. The assistant coaches were down in the pits with us. They, too, were afraid of him.

We lined up and ran the ball behind the right offensive guard. *Oh, no.* The defense stopped us again. We did not score.

From Coach Bryant's tower, a voice no less powerful than thunder commanded, "Get on the line." (That meant to line up and get ready to run a play). The protective chain at the top of the tower's ladder was snapped open (a sound that each player and assistant coach recognized and feared).

I was the offensive center. As I reached out for the football, I lowered my head and looked back through my legs only to see Coach Bryant come down the ladder as quickly as a fireman answering an alarm. When his boots hit the ground, he broke into a gallop heading toward the offensive line. By now each player was already down in his ready position. I could hear his feet pounding the ground as he came thundering toward us. I prayed again, "Dear God, don't let it be me."

Each player had his rear end set up as a target. He ran past the fullback, pushing him aside, and planted his left foot directly behind me. I cringed! Then Coach kicked the right offensive guard in the vulnerable spot, sending him tumbling into the end zone.

"Now," he said, "See if you can score. Run the same play." Needless to say, that time the offensive line blew the defense off the line of scrimmage. The runner made it into the end zone, untouched. This time, we were given a second chance, and succeeded. Second chances, as I later learned, aren't always available. A lesson had been learned. Fatigue is no excuse for non-performance.

On that particular April afternoon during spring training everyone survived the "gut-check." That was not always the case.

Those That Remained

But this was a new day. We anticipated another test. Could each of us do it again? That question was paramount in our minds. There was one thing in our favor. The temperature on Monday nights in October is not 102°. However, in that early morning "re-dedication" meeting, Coach Bryant was "hot." That could off-set the cooler weather.

When time approached to go to practice, each one of us went as though it might be our last trip to the athletic facilities at The University of Alabama. We anticipated an old-fashioned "gut-check," in which at least one or more players would be singled out to be pushed to the brink to see if they might decide to quit on the spot. No one knew whose number would be up.

What a shock! Practice that night was no different from any other Monday practice, except that several of our former teammates did not report. Coach Bryant had used the tactic of fear to cause each one of us to search deep into our own souls and see how important football was to us. He was testing us. Knowing that we might have to face difficult physical and mental circumstances that day, those of us who showed up to practice proved to him and to ourselves that we were willing to do whatever was required in order to help ourselves become a better player and to help our team have a chance to win. We had made our choice.

The Plan Revealed

Coach Bryant was a worrier and a realist, but when it came to believing that people can affect their destiny, if they do what they are capable of doing, he was the eternal optimist. Just prior to leaving for summer vacation before the 1964 season, he called the entire squad together and told us that he wanted to discuss the future.

He began the meeting by comparing football to life. He said, "One day you will find yourself in deep trouble—maybe you will have lost your job or business and be covered up with mortgages and debts. Your wife and children will look to you for leadership and guidance. What are you going to do? Will you feel sorry for yourself and blame others for your situation or will you get up off your rear ends and go to work? Maybe you will need two jobs or maybe you will have to create a job if one does not exist. The way you respond to adversity here at Alabama will determine how you will handle similar situations when you are out in the world on your own."

I believe that the way young people approach their work while in school is an early indication of how they will fare in adulthood with business, family and interpersonal relationships. Coach often talked to us as a father or counselor. Even today, when I am faced with a dilemma, I still reflect upon statements he made more than 20 years ago. He was preparing us for life after football. During those years I had less than ten one-on-one, face to face, private conversations with him, but each time he spoke to the squad, our eyes were fixed on his every gesture. He searched our eyes as though he was looking into our souls. Eyes don't lie.

Later, during that same meeting, he told us that he had been looking ahead to next season, and was convinced that our 1964 team could be National Champions if we *really* wanted to be and were willing to pay the price of victory.

It only takes 14-21 days of vigorous training for an athlete to whip his body into shape. It takes much longer to program the mind into becoming a winner. Deep in the subconscious mind, there is a factor called the "belief level." What we believe we can do, we can do. If we feel we are inferior, we will be. The primary reason for training is to program the belief level. The purpose of a "gut-check" is to get one to reach deep down and search for himself in the belief level. All the players at that meeting had passed the test. Coach Bryant knew it, and so did we.

He went to the blackboard and outlined a plan for us, step by step, telling us that both the coaches and players would first have to be totally committed toward being champions and that we would have to prepare ourselves during the summer break in order to achieve it. It would mean more than one hundred people working together to accomplish the same goal in order to get the job done. On the field we would not think as individuals, but as one. He called this phenomenon "Oneness." It proved to be the key to team success.

It was easy to see that he believed in us and that he was convinced that we could do it, together. We left that meeting with the confidence that he could lead us to the National Championship.

CHAPTER 7

A CHARACTER ASSASSINATION

In the early '60's, the University of Alabama usually opened its season against the University of Georgia. All spring and summer, we worked toward getting ready to "play Georgia." I did not realize, at that time, how fierce the competition was between the two states. It seems that the Georgia and Georgia Tech games created more controversy over the years than did the Alabama vs. Auburn games.

When the day came for us to play the University of Georgia, the game was played at Legion Field in Birmingham. We were prepared, but no more so than any other year nor for any other big game. Alabama had a good team that year (we went on to win the national championship) and Georgia had somewhat of an off-year, for it. The game was uneventful from our standpoint. We won it handily 32-6 and were off to a good start in achieving our goal.

Some sportswriters obviously took the outcome of that game with difficulty. There had been some bad blood between two universities (*Georgia Tech* and Alabama) and the media in each state. Apparently, a number of powerful media people decided to go after Coach Bryant. As I have learned more recently, some people resent the accomplishments of others and will go to ANY extreme to try to hurt someone who has achieved more success than some self-appointed "judges" think one deserves. The *Saturday Evening Post* published an article criticizing Coach Bryant and accusing him of teaching "brutality" to his players.

There had been an incident a few years previously in which a Georgia Tech player suffered a fractured jaw during an attempted block by an Alabama player on a punt. Much was and had been made by the Atlanta press about that incident. The *Post* article made accusations that were unfounded and clearly intended to hurt Coach Bryant, personally and professionally. In doing so, they would surely damage the image of the entire Alabama football program.

Shortly thereafter, a second article appeared, falsely accusing Coach Bryant and the former University of Georgia coach, Wally Butts, of "fixing" the 1962 Alabama vs. Georgia game, which we had won, 32-6. Georgia players were allegedly quoted in the article saying that we (Alabama) knew Georgia's plays, and often called them out before they were run.

Anyone who has followed football knows that after two schools have played for several years, each side develops a detailed scouting report prior to the next game. I'm sure Georgia had a scouting report on us. A team's offensive and defensive formations remain essentially the same and most teams develop tendencies or habits, running certain plays from certain formations in certain areas of the field on certain downs.

Football, like chess, is a game of probabilities. Today, computers are used to develop game plans and scouting reports. In the 1960s, Coach Bryant was a human computer. He was good at what he did and had achieved success in somewhat of an unconventional manner—he out-worked his opponents. Even though some considered him an "uneducated" man in the traditional sense, he outsmarted his adversaries. His success apparently made some people so envious that they would apparently go to *any* extreme to try to mar his reputation. At least they tried.

Kangaroo Court

The second *Saturday Evening Post* article was entitled, "The Story Of A College Football Fix." The *Post's* investigative team or kangaroo court attempted to "try" and convict both Coach Bryant and Coach Butts in that story. Neither of those men had reached their levels of success by letting others take advantage of them. They chose to fight back. They took the issue to the people. They sued and won. Both received substantial financial verdicts for punitive damages against their accusers, but, more importantly, they cleared their names and preserved the reputations that had taken lifetimes of hard work to establish.

Truth Prevailed

The credibility of his accusers fell to an all-time low. Shortly thereafter, the *Saturday Evening Post* went out of business. Truth prevailed. In the end, it always does.

Coach Bryant did what he had to do to protect his reputation. I know he would advise me and anyone else to do the same if he were alive today. Irresponsible people must answer for their malicious deeds. I feel that the attacks on Coach Bryant and the manner in which he handled the situation gave strength and commitment to our team that year. As we learned on many occasions, adversity often is the stimulus needed to extract greatness from mediocrity.

CHAPTER 8

IN PURSUIT OF THE CHAMPIONSHIP

"They can because
They think they can."[1]

When our players returned to The University of Alabama campus in mid-August prior to the 1964 season, the temperature had been in the high 90s. Tuscaloosa always seemed the hottest spot in the state. During one of our early meetings, Coach Bryant reviewed our plans and had a chart of our upcoming schedule placed on our dressing room wall so that each game could be marked off, one by one. As the weeks went by, we steadfastly got closer to our goal.

One autumn Saturday afternoon, we returned to Atlanta to play Georgia Tech. Those of us who had been there two years previously had waited for that day. We were anxious to have an opportunity to play Tech again. Once more, for Alabama, the national championship would be on the line. This time, we were dedicated to coming away with a different verdict. Some of us would have a second chance, this time.

The first half of the game was a knock-down, drag-out affair just

---

[1]Virgil, *Motivational Quotes* p. 47.

as it had been two years previously. With 90 seconds remaining in the first half, the score was still 0-0. Joe Namath was injured and had not played. During a timeout, we looked up and saw him jogging onto the field, on his "fragile" knee.

As he stepped into the huddle, he told us that he had been studying the Tech defensive backs and felt that they were vulnerable. He felt that we would need to run a couple of running plays to "set up" the touchdown pass and explained to each man in the huddle what each of us needed to do. On the third play he said, "It is set up perfectly. You guys, (the offensive line) give me the time to throw the pass and you (the receiver) catch the ball, and we've got a touchdown!" Six seconds later, just as he had predicted, the score was Alabama 6, Georgia Tech 0.

We lined up for the kick-off and went for an on-sides kick. Sure enough, we recovered the ball and the stage was set again. A second time, Namath outlined a plan for a touchdown. Needless to say, our confidence level was high. We thought we could do it again. As he predicted, within seconds, the second touchdown was scored. Success breeds success.

Within 90 seconds, our team had scored two touchdowns. At half-time we led 14-0. We went on to win the game and avenge a painful loss which had occurred on that same field two years previously. This time it was Coach Bryant who was met at midfield to be congratulated; however, the Tech coach didn't come to our dressing room to congratulate our team. The dressing room scene in Atlanta that afternoon was quite different. As one might anticipate by now, Coach Bryant gave all of the credit for the victory to his players and assistant coaches and told the press that the only plays he called during the game were the ones that didn't work. We all knew the true story, however. Success begins at the top—planning, organizing, motivating, and evaluating. That's how one controls his destiny.

The Iron Bowl

Each week we were able to check off the victories on the chart in our practice dressing room until only the "big one" remained. In Alabama, it is referred to as "The Iron Bowl," the state championship between Alabama and Auburn played in Birmingham's Legion Field. In 1964, both schools had good teams, so the game was to be nationally televised and played in Birmingham on Thanksgiving Day. Many of the Alabama players had friends on the Auburn squad, some were former teammates from high school and all-star games. We had followed their careers during college and they ours.

In Alabama, football is more than a sport. For many, it seems to be a way of life. After the 1984 Alabama victory over Auburn (17-15), Coach Ray Perkins said, "The game seems to be more important to the fans than I had ever recognized as a player."

The outcome of the Alabama-Auburn game seems to affect social events in the state. I have observed that when Alabama wins the Iron Bowl, more Alabama fans seem to come out to certain social events (Touchdown and Quarterback Club meetings). When Auburn wins, some of the same people stay home and more Auburn fans seem to turn out. I know of no other state where so much rides on the outcome of a single game.

On Thanksgiving Day, 1964, Legion Field was packed with people wearing Auburn's blue and orange and Alabama's red and white. The stadium trembled with "Roll Tide" and "War Eagle" as each cheering section carried out their own battles in the stands. At halftime, the score was Auburn 7, Alabama 6. In the dressing room, Coach Bryant said, "We've got them right where we want them. Now, let's go out there and do what we came here to do." I thought, "How do we have "them right where we want them? We are behind 7-6."

He certainly convinced Raymond Ogden, the halfback who was to receive the kick-off, that we had them where we wanted them. In the huddle, before the opening kick-off of the second half, Ogden said, "Just let me get the ball and don't anybody get in my path, 'cause I'm going to take this one all the way."

My responsibility on the kick-off return play was to block the kicker as he came running down the field. He kicked seven yards deep in the end zone. Ogden had already told us his plans. He caught the ball and started up the field. I blocked the kicker as directed and rolled over to see where Ogden was. He was running straight toward me, so I got up quickly and headed down field again in front of him. At that time, I saw another Auburn player out of the corner of my eye and tried to get in his way. Fortunately, as I threw the block, he fell over me. As he was going down, we realized that we knew each other well and exchanged comments. He was Bill Edge, now a surgeon in Birmingham. (Bill had been to my home in Enterprise several times while visiting the girl he eventually married. We had also been out together following previous Alabama vs. Auburn games.) As I looked up again, all 200 pounds of Raymond Ogden's frame were galloping toward the Auburn end zone to score what turned out to be the touchdown that turned things around and sealed the dream outlined five months previously by Coach Bryant.

Going into that Alabama-Auburn game, Joe Namath needed only a few more yards to surpass the all-time Alabama passing record. Toward the end of the game, one or two completions could have given Joe the new record, but he chose not to put the ball into the air. To him, winning the game for his team and his school was more important than individual glory. The record was certainly his for the taking. He knew it and so did we. Namath was a *team* player. That's only one of the traits that made him one of the greatest "giants" the game of football ever produced.

The 1964 Alabama team needed the help of Notre Dame the following Saturday to seal the National Championship. It upset Southern Cal, who was ahead of us in the polls, in a fourth quarter comeback win. When the votes were counted on Monday, Alabama came out on top. We were No. 1. Our pre-conceived destiny was a

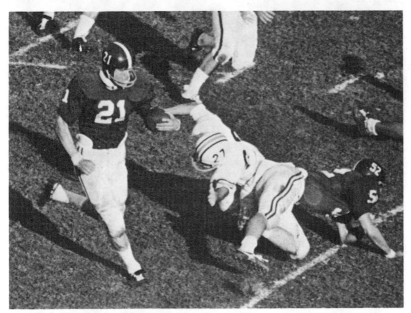

Raymond Ogden runs for a TD against Auburn on Thanksgiving Day, 1964. Gaylon McCollough (52) blocks Auburn safety man, Bill Edge (27).

reality. We had earned it based upon the plan established by Coach Bryant and adopted by our team almost seven months previously.

I'll never forget where I was when Coach Bryant broke the news to us. I was eating lunch in Bryant Hall (the living quarters for Alabama athletes) with Joe Namath, Ray Perkins and Raymond Ogden.

A photographer was there and captured a moment of history.

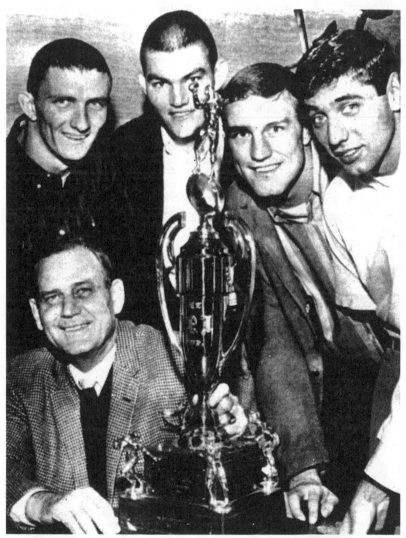

Coach Bryant with Ray Perkins, Raymond Ogden, Gaylon McCollough and Joe Namath celebrating the 1964 National Championship.

The Guarantee Fulfilled

One of the most memorable days in my life was when the gold and diamond national championship rings arrived for each of the players, coaches and staff of that 1964 team. Four years previously, Coach Bob Ford had sat at the breakfast table of my home when I was trying to make the decision about my football future. As I placed the ring on my hand, I could almost hear Coach Ford's comments to me. "If you want to go to college and win a lot of games and have some fun, go on over to Georgia Tech, but if you want one of these (rings), come on to Alabama and *I guarantee you, you will own one before you leave there.*" I still wear that ring. What it stands for becomes more important to me with each passing year. The ring serves as a reminder that anything is possible, even against insurmountable odds. For that group of scrappy players averaging 185 pounds per man and coming from all walks of life to have emerged as "the nation's best" was a tribute to our parents, hometowns, teachers, coaches, and all who believed in the University of Alabama's program. The Championship belonged to all those who shared in the lives of each player, and to the giants of the past who helped establish the "Alabama Tradition."

We did it because
We believed we could.
As one, we climbed upon
The shoulders of giants.

1964 NATIONAL CHAMPIONS Alabama Crimson Tide

Alabama 31, Georgia 3

Alabama 36, Tulane 6

Alabama 24, Vanderbilt 0

Alabama 21, N. C. State 0

Alabama 19, Tennessee 8

Alabama 17, Florida 14

Alabama 23, Miss. State 6

Alabama 17, L. S. U. 9

Alabama 24, Georgia Tech 7

Alabama 21, Auburn 14

Head Coach Paul Bryant

1964 CRIMSON TIDE SQUAD—SOUTHEASTERN CONFERENCE CHAMPIONS

Front row, left to right: David Ray, John Williams, Jerry Duncan, John Calvert, Creed Gilmer, Dudley Kerr, John Mosley, Wayne Trimble, Leslie Kelley, Robert Rumsey, Dickie Bean, Harold Moore, John Sullivan.

Second row, l to r: Ron Durby, Larry Wall, Joe Namath, Mike Hopper, Jim Simmons, Raymond Ogden, Gaylon McCollough, Mickey Andrews, Charlie Stephens, Kenneth Mitchell, Frankie McClendon, Hudson Harris, Buddy French, Dan Keenley, Ron Bird, Wayne Freeman.

Back row, l to r: Cecil Dowdy, Steve Sloan, Bill Tugwell, Wayne Cook, Vernon Newbill, Paul Crane, Tim Bates, Ray Perkins, Tommy Tolleson, Ben McLeod, Lynn Strickland, Jim Fuller, Richard Cole, Jimmy Carroll, Steve Bowman, Louis Thompson. Missing: Jackie Sherrill, Grady Elmore and Frank Canterbury.

CHAPTER 9

A PROFESSIONAL COWBOY...ALMOST

*"We are continually faced
by great opportunities
Brilliantly disguised as
insoluble problems."*[1]

During the 1964 season, I had been contacted by several professional football teams, but when the Dallas Cowboys called, all the others went to second place. What small boy didn't play cowboys and indians and idolize the heroes of the old west who sat tall in the saddle? I guess the boy in me wanted to be a grown-up cowboy in Texas. In addition, one of my former teammates and roommate on Alabama road trips, Lee Roy Jordan, was playing for the Cowboys. The thought of, once again, establishing the Jordan (defense)-McCollough (offense) Alabama connection was appealing and challenging.

When the Cowboys started talking about signing bonuses and salaries for playing football, this 'ole boy from Enterprise, Alabama began to listen, and listen hard. There was a problem, however. I had taken a pre-medical school curriculum (that is one of the reasons that

---

[1]Anonymous, *Motivational Quotes* p. 67.

I had chosen the University of Alabama) and had already applied to medical school in Birmingham. Actually, pro football had never been one of my dreams. It certainly had not been part of my career planning, but it was a great opportunity—a chance I hadn't anticipated.

The possibility of going to medical school during the off season while under contract with the Cowboys was an exciting option, but would take time, time that I didn't have. I had not even applied to the medical schools which allowed such a plan. The application process to medical school is a lengthy and complex affair, often taking months to complete with no assurance for acceptance.

Still, the option was there for the taking. The more I considered the glamour and the financial rewards for pro football, the more appealing it became. I would also go to medical school, somewhere.

A great deal of arm-twisting had already been done at Alabama's medical school to help me get accepted immediately following graduation. Because of football practice, however, I had not been able to take some of the pre-requisite laboratory courses. It had been suggested that I wait a year, so that I could get these subjects behind me. Retrospectively, the admission people probably were right. I had already learned that anything is possible if one has a goal and is willing to work and I told the medical school registrar so.

Later, the admissions committee agreed to take a chance on me, so I had a "bird in the hand."

The Dallas Cowboy organization is and has been a most impressive outfit. The monetary carrot got bigger and bigger with each passing week and the temptation to play, even for a while, was certainly appealing. I needed to talk to someone about this professional football business.

Namath's Game

Joe Namath and I had become "pool-shooting buddies". After the 1964 season we frequently went downtown in Tuscaloosa after dinner for an hour or so to play a few games at The Shamrock.

He was in the midst of big-time negotiations with both the New York Jets of the AFL and the St. Louis Cardinals of the NFL. One night, I told him that the Cowboy organization and I were also talking business. All of this was new to me, and I asked if he would give me some idea of how much professional teams paid their players; furthermore, would he mind telling me what the Jets and Cardinals were offering him so that I could have some idea of what to ask for.

He said, "Gaylon, I just talked to my attorney and he told me that today's offer was around $200,000."

"What?" I asked in amazement, "Joe, you are joking, aren't you? I will be the first to admit that you are a GREAT player, but I can't see how any player can be worth that much money."

"My lawyer tells me that we are just getting started," Joe added.

He was right. Within the next few weeks, Joe would become the highest paid football player to play the game, up to that time. In the end, the New York Jets and the American Football League got a bargain in the deal. He, more than any other player, established the credibility of the AFL which led to the merger with the NFL.

Joe Namath is a living example of the American dream. He came from the streets of Beaver Falls, Pennsylvania where he and his childhood friend, Jimmy, walked, pulling their wagon filled with returnable soft drink bottles. He made it to the streets of Broadway where he was escorted in long black limousines.

Joe Namath never backed down from a challenge, and even when the odds appeared to be against him, he transcended adversity in his own inimitable style: from the crippled quarterback carried off the field in 1963 on a stretcher at Bryant-Denny Stadium in Tuscaloosa, to the Super Bowl Champion carried off the field in Miami on the shoulders of his Jet teammates; and from the unpolished motorcycle kid he played in a movie early in his acting career, to the dynamic, debonaire Sky Masterson of "Guys and Dolls."

Joe has been successful because he has a great capacity to comprehend, analyze and produce.

To those who have had the opportunity to know the man and see him grow, he has been much more:

— a face you were glad to see at the other end of a huddle on third-and-15 when you were behind in the fourth quarter,

— an adopted nephew to three little ladies from Tuscaloosa who gave him a home away from home (They were his special guests when he was inducted into Alabama's Sports Hall of Fame),

— a devoted friend to Jack (Hootowl) Hicks, one of his partners in the purchase of his first automobile, a four-door 1953 Ford that had no doors,

— a son, who rather than spending it on himself, sent ticket money

home to his mother and sister while he was in college.
— a kind, considerate, polite man with good manners who never out-
grew his friends and wears his American heritage with pride.

Football was Joe's game. It became his profession. For me, it was
a different story.

Logic Prevails

The NATIONAL CHAMPION ALABAMA CRIMSON TIDE was
set to play Southwest Conference Champion, Texas, in the Orange
Bowl on New Year's Eve, 1964, the first time the game was played
at night. In those days, fortunately, for us, the national championship
was awarded prior to the bowl games. On the way to Miami, my
thoughts were occupied by several factors which were about to affect
my future: the Longhorns, the Cowboys, medical school, and Miss
Alabama, not necessarily in that order, however.

My parents, who still live in Enterprise, had never been to Miami,
nor had they flown in an airplane. The Cowboy organization offered
to arrange for them to go to Miami and pay their expenses while
there. That's legal. For that opportunity, I shall always be grateful to
the Dallas Cowboy organization and to Delta Airlines, which helped
us get my mother and father home during the holiday rush following
the game.

Looking back, however, the fact that my father was in Miami that
week may have been a key factor in the decision not to accept the
Cowboys' offer. Maybe they, too, should be grateful to him.

While standing in the lobby of our hotel one day that week, my
father met a loyal Alabama fan in Miami. Dr. Ellis Porch practices
medicine in Arab, Alabama, and had followed the Alabama team all
over the country. He still does.

Following a conversation with Dr. Porch, my dad came looking for
me. When he found me, he said, "I just met a man you need to talk
with."

I did. Dr. Porch told me that he had heard the facts from my dad
and that at my father's request, he was going to give me some advice. He proceeded to tell me what it meant to him to be a physician
and outlined the risks of serious injury while playing pro football. He
also discussed the possibility of getting wrapped up in "the good life"
which would be available with the money one would receive while

playing. With the temptation not to give up the "good life" I might get sidetracked. He said it would also be very tempting to continue to delay going to medical school and that I just might get distracted and decide not to complete medical school. The longer it took for me to get my M.D. degree, the less likely I would be to go on and specialize.

"Specialization" he said, "will become more important in the coming years. I am a general practitioner. Already, I can see the benefits of specialization for your generation." Every time I see Dr. Ellis Porch, I feel the need to thank him for being in Miami that week.

During that period, I received advice from many people, sometimes unsolicited. One day I opened a letter from my former high school principal and neighbor, Oscar Zeanah. It was short and to the point, as Mr. Zeanah usually was. It read, "Dear Gaylon, Boys play football." He knew *my game* should be a medical career.

After thinking about his words, it occurred to me that sooner or later, every athlete must lay aside that part of his life and come face to face with the real world. An athlete's fame is short-lived. There is always someone younger, bigger, stronger and faster closing in on his job. The end of his career is only one play, or one injury away, at any given time. Athletics, I have learned, should be used as a training ground or steppingstone into a more permanent lifetime career. Too many athletes are at the peak of their careers while playing. That's not how it should be. The failure to take advantage of an education is an opportunity wasted.

My parents had told me that one's education is forever and that an educational degree could be a ticket for lasting success. Call it job security.

After considering my options, I realized that I did not have a problem but a "great opportunity." I had a choice. My fate to become a facial surgeon had been "brilliantly disguised as an insoluble problem."

Looking back, I now know that I made the right decision, but I often wonder: "Wouldn't it have been interesting to have been a Cowboy for a while? What would destiny have held for me? What would my life be like today had I made a different choice?"

Who knows. . . .?

CHAPTER 10

NO SECOND CHANCE

Miss Alabama, Susan Nomberg, was in New York during the Christmas holidays visiting some of her family, but I knew she would be watching the 1964 Orange Bowl game on television.

The Cowboy representative was in the press box, the Longhorns team was on the opposite side of the field, and the president of the United States, Lyndon Johnson, a Texan, was sitting in the stands behind the Longhorn bench. Everyone was ready for an old-fashioned shoot-out. Anybody looking for excitement was not to be disappointed. Jackie Gleason came to the center of the field for the toss of the coin following which he exclaimed, "Away we go."

The Texas Longhorns obviously came to Miami for an ambush and brought plenty of ammunition. Anyone wanting to know "where's the beef?" that night could have looked on the Longhorn's sidelines and easily found it. They were big, strong, and fast: a herd of bulls.

A Game Has Two Halves

The first half of the game belonged to Texas. Then, at halftime, as we had done so many times during the past four years, our team regrouped and the coaching staff adjusted the game plan.

Once again, a crippled Joe Namath would come into the game and turn things around. Changing our offensive scheme and passing on first and second downs, we rallied and made the score Texas 21, Alabama 17 with about three minutes left in the game.

After a long drive, the ball was resting on the two yard line. We had second down and goal to go for a come-from-behind touchdown. Once again, the "cardiac kids" looked as if though they were going to pull the game out. The "sizzling seven" offensive linemen (Wayne Cook, Frankie McClendon, Wayne Freeman, Gaylon McCollough, Tank Mitchell, Ron Derby and Ray Perkins) were in for a challenge.

What was to follow would be the most memorable three plays of my entire football career. Three plays that would help shape the remainder of my life—a glimpse of destiny.

We had not been able to run the ball effectively against the big Texas defensive line all night, but surely, we would make two yards in three plays. If we couldn't, we didn't deserve to win.

Two plunges into the line took the ball to the one foot line. On fourth down, Namath called a quarterback sneak with wedge blocking. That means the entire offensive line blocks toward a spot between the center and the right guard.

As we went to the line of scrimmage, every member of our team assumed that we would score the touchdown and win the game. I certainly did.

I reached out for the ball resting twelve inches away from the end zone, twelve inches from another comeback win with the President of the United States and 70,000 other fans in the stands. Most of sports America and Miss Alabama were watching on television.

Dyrone Talbert was the outstanding Texas defensive lineman who had been giving me a tough time all night. He was lined up right in the spot the play was to be run, between the right guard (Wayne Freeman) and me. Our offensive blocking rule dictated that I help Freeman block him.

Just as the play was to begin, the All-American Texas (and later, Atlanta Falcon) linebacker, Tommy Nobis, rushed to the line of scrimmage and lined up right on my nose. I had to make a decision, quickly. Was I to block my designated assignment or use my judgement, and try to block Nobis, who certainly would reach out and grab Joe if I didn't block him? In the bat of an eye, Joe gave the signal to me to snap the ball to him and the two lines crashed into each other like 14 bulls, straining and twisting for all we were worth.

When the play was over, I looked for Namath. It was easy to find him. He was lying on top of me *in the end zone*. We jumped up and began to celebrate. One official indicated "TOUCHDOWN!!" The line judge came running toward the pile and asked, "Did he score?" "Yes" the first official replied. Then, suddenly, the bottom fell out. The head official came running from behind, quickly took the ball from the one who had first indicated a touchdown, placed the ball just short of the goal line and indicated "first down" for Texas. NO TOUCHDOWN!!!

We could not believe what had just happened. Although we protested, it was to no avail. The initial touchdown indication was overruled and the score remained Texas 21, Alabama 17.

A Margin of Safety

Feeling both anger and persecution, the offensive team headed to the sideline. That trip to our bench was the longest I had ever taken in a football game. I guess we all looked straight at Coach Bryant. Where had he been through all of the confusion? Standing there on the sideline. He knew that the decision would not be reversed. It was over.

I thought of the "gut-check" in the spring of 1962, when we were given a second chance, and scored. This time, there would be no second chance. Someone said to him as he walked past, "Coach, we scored." He continued looking straight ahead and replied, "If he (Joe) had walked in [to the end zone with a football], there could have been no question about it."

He always knew the right words to say in any situation. He taught us one final lesson right on the spot. If you want to accomplish something, don't do just enough to try to get the job done. Go beyond what is required. Leave a margin of safety and don't rely upon other people to judge success or failure in ourselves. Life is not always fair, so it is up to each of us to get the job done, beyond questions.

Opportunity Knocked Once

Did I make an error in judgement? Was I wrong to block Nobis instead of Talbert? If I had the chance to do it over again, what would I do differently? In life, we don't usually get a second chance either. Planning and preparation beforehand then executing at that important moment converts a near miss to success. If I had made a different choice, would the outcome have been different?

This much I do know. We can't go back in time. Opportunity knocked once. If I could have had a second chance on that goal line in the Orange Bowl, I believe that I would have made a better block. I think my teammates would have too, and we would have won, without question. I learned something that night. Ever since, I have tried to leave no room for doubt. I am still trying to score that one that didn't happen. I believe it has been a driving force in my life and has helped me achieve more of my own personal goals since.

The seniors on that 1964 team lost the last game we ever played for Alabama. Even though we lost only four games during the four years we played there, we let the University down on that particular night in Miami. I guess we took all the victories for granted. Winning had become a habit. We never went into a game wondering IF we would win. The question in our minds was by how much would we win and would we play well.

We did learn from those four losses, however. Each one was always used as a steppingstone for next week. After that 1964 Orange Bowl game, there wasn't a "next" game for most of our seniors. The next game was the game of life.

That goal line experience in Miami drives me today to become a better man and to do any job to the best of my ability—I might not get a second chance.

CHAPTER 11

MISS ALABAMA

During the fall of 1962, a calendar was published by The University of Alabama spotlighting its new "Miss Alabama," Susan Nomberg, from Dothan. The moment I saw her picture, I thought, "this is the most beautiful creature I have ever seen." It was easy to find out who she was and where she lived, so I called her up to ask her if she would go out with me. She didn't know me from any of the other guys who called, but she was polite and thanked me for the invitation.

I was persistent and called back several other times, but continued to get turned down. Over the next two years, I continued to call her. During summer vacation, when I visited Dothan, (30 miles from Enterprise), I called her. Her father always screened her calls and I never seemed to be able to "catch her at home." I was beginning to develop a complex.

Fate finally took over. In the fall of 1964, I took a criminology course (Social Treatment of the Youthful Offender taught by Emory Hubbard). When I walked into the classroom and saw her there, I knew my luck was about to change. It did, and at last, she accepted the invitation for a date. From that time until today, we have been together. Later that year, we were married. In 1986, we celebrated our 21st consecutive wedding anniversary, a fact in which we both take great pride. So many people thought our marriage would surely fail

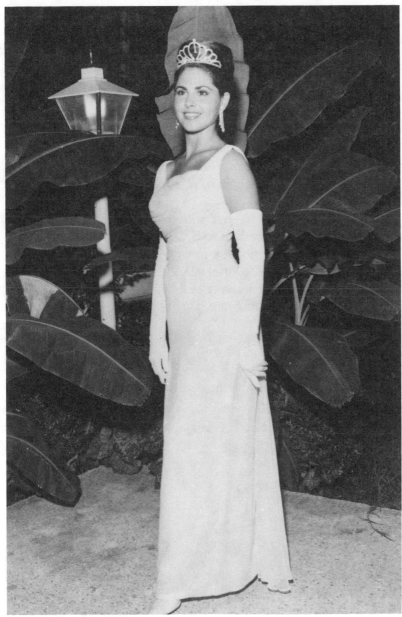

Susan Nomberg (McCollough), Miss Alabama, 1962.

because of our different backgrounds. It has worked, because we chose to make it work. Miss Alabama became Mrs. McCollough and with that opted to give up her own career to become a mother and my wife.

In *The Rebirth of America,* President Ronald Reagan acknowledged the family unit's contribution to our country's success.

"America's families make immeasurable contributions to America's well-being. Today, more than ever, it is essential that these contributions not be taken for granted and that each of us remembers that **the strength of our families is vital to the strength of our nation.**"[1]

Susan and I have been blessed with two wonderful children. Sted was born while I was in medical school. Blessed with talent and creativity, he is currently in the New College program at the University of Alabama in a pre-architectural curriculum. (Somehow that has a familiar ring.) During the summer of 1986, he attended the School of Architecture at Mississippi State. He has some decisions to make.

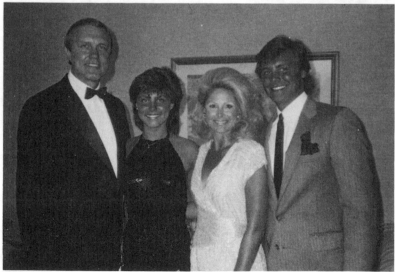

Dr. McCollough, Chanee, Susan, and Sted in 1986 at the spring meeting of the AAFPRS in Palm Beach, Fla.

---

[1]Everett Hale, *Rebirth of America* p. 97.

In the spring of 1986, Chanee earned the gold medal from the United States Figure Skating Association for successfully completing her eighth figure test. She trained in Atlanta, Lake Placid, and Los Angeles. Where she goes from here is a matter of choice, for her.

I often wonder what might have happened had I not signed up for that criminology class. Maybe fate would have taken another route to achieve this same end.

CHAPTER 12

FIRST, BECOME A DOCTOR

In August 1965, Susan and I moved from a small basement apartment in Tuscaloosa to a smaller concrete block apartment on Birmingham's Southside, behind South Highlands Hospital. Our parents had given us a few pieces of furniture from their homes to help us get started.

That first apartment in Birmingham required a full day of scrubbing down the walls and floors with Lysol disinfectant. We paid $49 per month for it. That was too much.

At the end of my college career, my hometown honored me with "Gaylon McCollough Day." The citizens of Enterprise gave me $1,000 to be used toward my education. With my parents' help and a federal student loan of about $1,200.00, we got by that first year just fine. We didn't know anybody else was doing any better. We thought all the other couples were in the same boat. Retrospectively, I believe it is good to "do without" many of the things we want or think we need. When one works his way up, he generally appreciates what he gets more than if it was given to him on a silver platter.

Medical school was every bit as tough as the registrar, Virginia Baxley, told me it was going to be. We usually went to class and labs about 8 hours each day or 40 hours per week. In addition, I studied for at least 6 hours each night after class and during most of the day on Saturday and Sunday.

I had learned that the way to increase one's capacity was to exhaust one's self—to go further than the day before. The mind's capacity is astounding. It is greater than that of a modern computer twice the size of the Empire State Building. Although I had successfully survived Coach Bryant's physical "gut-checks," I had never before been academically challenged, at least not to the extent that I faced that first month in medical school.

Susan and I managed to go out for a spaghetti dinner on our first anniversary and I attended a couple of Alabama football games. I was too scared to take time away from my studies. I had to pass. The commitment had been made. I must become a doctor. Too much was riding on my successfully completing that first year.

A Small Cheering Section

On Sunday afternoons, we would turn on our little black and white television set that Max and Dottie (Susan's parents) had given us so that we could watch my former teammates play pro football. Between plays and during commercials, I would study my anatomy book and think of what might have been had I decided to become a Dallas Cowboy. During those days, I second-guessed myself hundreds of times. I must admit that I missed the excitement of game day, the crowd, the competition, and the recognition bestowed an athlete.

The salary offered by the Cowboys was another matter. I looked around our tiny apartment, furnished with second-hand furniture, and thought of how different things could have been in Dallas. Had I made the right choice? Was my destiny to become a physician? Could I make it happen?

I was starting all over again as a freshman in medical school, essentially isolated from the outside world. There was no team spirit. It was every student "scratching" to stay alive, academically, to make his grades. There was no coach assigned to me to evaluate my every move and help correct errors. The fanfare, color and excitement has been replaced with uncertainty and apprehension. I had gone from participating in a team sport to individual competition, like the ice skater, the gymnast or the track and field competitor. It was a whole new ball game. My cheering section had been reduced to Susan and our immediate families.

When my medical school class had its first set of exams, I was more apprehensive than before any football game in which I had played. Awaiting results of those exams was much like watching a Van Tiffin field goal, which would decide the outcome of an important game, head toward the goal posts. When the outcome of an event is so crucial to one's future, seconds seem like minutes, minutes like hours, hours like days.

The test scores were posted. We made it—I passed. Susan and I cheered, then celebrated with another spaghetti dinner. I was on my way. Getting by that first hurdle was a critical step. The work and study didn't get any easier but my confidence level was much higher and the self-imposed pressure was relieved. I discovered that medical school was really no different from any other challenge I had faced. Planning, organization, hard work, honesty and self-assessment are the keys to achieving any goal. A small cheering section helps.

Duke and Mimi

Later that year when Sted was on the way, we moved away from that little apartment to a small frame house behind Idlewild Circle. Our next-door neighbors were Duke ("The Duke") and Mimi Rumore, a long time Birmingham radio family. They were wonderful people, and looked after a young, naive married couple with a new baby during those two years.

My parents had borrowed money from a bank in Enterprise to buy that little house. The Hendersons took a chance on the McColloughs again, and my father signed the note. He let us move into the house once the loan was secured.

Susan and I made furniture out of old doors, boards and concrete blocks, then tried to dye the carpet to change its color. (What a mess! That was one of the worst ideas I ever had.) My mother made curtains for us. Max, my father-in-law, and I repainted the house. It was truly a team project from both sides of our families, but we had a plan and didn't mind a little inconvenience and work. It was the best we could do at the time, so we accepted what was and dreamed of what might come.

After Sted was born, Susan went to work at Glen Iris Elementary School teaching special education children. I went to work at Lloyd Noland Hospital at night and on weekends in surgery as an operating room technician. During that time, we developed so many wonderful friendships which have provided advice, love and understanding along the way. Duke and Mimi, Martha and Gus Smith, Jim and Becky Thompson and Luna and Lee Hudson—"Thanks."

Each of these people shored us up by his or her friendship during difficult years. To have had one friend would have been enough; eight was a windfall.

My First Face Lift

It became obvious that we needed a second car, so I went looking. I bought an 18-year old Chevy for $60 from a gas station near our house. It was in terrible shape. I gave it a new paint job with a paint brush and two quarts of black enamel paint. It was an interesting experience getting back and forth across town to Lloyd Noland Hospital in that old car. There was no I-59 interstate then. The gears would lock-up at stop lights and traffic jams, so I carried a large wrench with me in order to "unlock them." The floor of the car was rusted out and the muffler had a large hole in it, therefore, I could not drive with the windows up, even in the winter or when it rained; otherwise, I would run the risk of carbon monoxide poisoning.

The car's battery was so bad that I had to park on an incline so that I could push the car off to crank it. My dad referred to that 1948 Chevy as an "accident looking for a place to happen."

After a few months of work, we saved some money and got a loan from another small bank back home in South Alabama which enabled us to trade the old Chevy in for a newer, more reliable model. Interestingly, when I sold the car, I made $10 on the deal. I guess it was the face lift I gave it with the new paint job.

The Ellards

Two years later, we decided to trade the little house on Southside for one on Valley View Circle in Homewood. That's where we lived when Chanee, our daughter, was born. It was this move that helped establish a lifelong friendship between our family and our new nextdoor neighbors, The Ellards (Bill, Jean, Dru and Jennifer). Bill is the president of Ellard Contracting Company. I have learned much from watching him deal with the ups and downs of the construction industry and the unpredictability of the weather. Both of them can make or break a construction company. Lesser men than he would have folded long ago. "Gut-checks," I learned, occur in the business world, too. Through good times and bad, he has maintained his integrity and has kept life in perspective—not only because he's tall (6'9"), but because of the principles for which he stands, I consider him one of those giants from whom I have gained wisdom.

VIP House Call

Medical school was a lot of hard work and little play. When not in class or working at the University Hospital, I worked elsewhere. If a job wasn't available, I would try to create one. I had grown up working, thinking that was what anyone was supposed to do in one's spare time. I wanted my wife and children to have the things I thought we needed, and working was the only way I knew to get them.

One of my more interesting work experiences came when I was hired to screen medical problems for guests at Birmingham's Parliament House (now the Holiday Inn-Medical Center). Early one morning the hotel operator called me at home and said that one of the VIP guests needed a doctor. When the voice on the other end of the phone said, "Doc, this is Roy Orbison" (a popular entertainer of the day), I thought it must be a prank. After talking with the man on the other end of the line, I became convinced that he was Roy Orbison. At 4 a.m., I dressed and went to the hotel. The desk clerk told me that Mr. Orbison was in the penthouse suite. I went there and knocked. He opened the door and told me that he was having "another" kidney stone attack. Most people know that kidney stone attacks often require injections of narcotics. I must admit I was suspicious about his story, and recommended that we contact a "real" doctor about having him admitted to South Highland's Hospital. When he quickly agreed, I realized that, indeed, he must have a kidney stone. At the hospital, his diagnosis was confirmed. I owed Roy Orbison an apology for doubt. I had jumped to a conclusion without knowing the facts. It was a good lesson for a doctor-in-training.

Time Out For Professional Football

During my junior year in medical school, I received another call from the Parliament House. This time, it was from one of its owners, Jim Lane. He wanted me to meet him for dinner at the hotel to discuss "a business proposition." In those days, I didn't turn down many steak dinners, so I went to hear what Mr. Lane had to say. He told me that the NFL had established a farm system, much like major league baseball had, and that he and the Atlanta Falcon organization had agreed to put a team in Huntsville, Alabama.

Most of the players would be promising young prospects who were working their way up to the NFL. Many of my college teammates and friends would be playing in this new league. The (Huntsville) "Alabama Hawks" had most every position covered except offensive center and he wanted me to come and play with them. I had already turned down an opportunity to play professional football in the big leagues and told Mr. Lane, "No thanks." He was persistent and insisted that I come up to Huntsville and at least look at their program. So, I drove up there and found many of my former teammates from Alabama and friends from Auburn, Georgia and other top schools on the practice field.

One of my former Enterprise High teammates, Jim Dyar, had played at the University of Houston and had been drafted by the Atlanta Falcons. Jim had been an outstanding defensive tackle in college, but did not possess the necessary size to play defensive tackle in the NFL. He did, however, have the speed and the strength necessary to be an offensive guard, so this was a perfect opportunity for him to get a year's experience before challenging NFL veteran guards or rookies with four years of college experience at that position.

I was impressed with the Huntsville organization and the thought of renewing some old friendships was appealing. Mr. Lane and I talked money. He offered me $150.00 per game, a far cry from what The Cowboys had offered, but more money than I made for an entire month's work at Lloyd Noland Hospital "moon-lighting" as a part-time operating room technician. He said he had offered the maximum salary that they could pay any player. I wanted to get the best deal possible, so I offered to play if I could also be an assistant to the team doctor as a trainer. I had not yet received my medical degree, so as

a medical student, I would have to work under the direction of a licensed physician. The Hawks agreed to pay me a total of $200.00
per game plus my expenses in getting back and forth from Birmingham. I chose to give football one more try. Maybe then I could get it
out of my system.

It was a two hour drive to Huntsville so I could not go there every
day to practice. I convinced them that, as an offensive center, I had
only four options on any given play—block straight ahead, block to
the right, block to the left or drop back and pass block. I would "work
out" in Birmingham every day and come to Huntsville to practice on
Thursday nights in order to learn any new plays put in for the game
on Saturday. They bought it, and I was playing football again. Each
weekend, Susan, Sted and "Bobo" (his stuffed monkey) traveled to
Huntsville with me to watch Daddy play football.

Fortunately, I was on an "elective" program that fall in medical
school. That meant that I had no night call or weekend responsibilities. The timing was perfect. It seemed as if everything was falling
in place again.

A Close Call

The season was fun and, surprisingly, it was a good brand of football and it was nice to be playing again. I had missed many aspects
of the game. We had a good team and played in the National Professional Football League's championship game, our "Super Bowl." At
the end of the season, I was named to the All-Pro Team as an offensive center.

Although we weren't playing in the NFL, many of the players from
the National Professional Football League of America did move up
the following year. Some had been called up during that same year for
a game or two or had played the previous year. The experience convinced me that I, too, could have made it with the Cowboys and that
realization got playing football out of my system.

I was lucky that I did not get seriously injured. I've often heard
that God looks after fools and small children. During our last regular
season game in Oklahoma, we played the Dallas Cowboy farm team
(ironic, huh?). I was covering a punt and got clipped. When I landed
on my back, I was paralyzed in the lower half of my body for about
30 seconds. As I laid there, on my back, I looked up beyond the stars

and prayed that I was not going to be permanently paralyzed. "Dear God?" I asked, "let me get up and walk across this field under my own power and when this season is over, I will never play football again." He answered that prayer and I went back to being a fulltime medical student again.

The Master Diagnostician

"No greater opportunity or obligation can fall the lot of a human being than to be a physician. In the care of the suffering he needs technical skill, scientific knowledge, and human understanding. He who uses these with courage, humility, and wisdom will provide a unique service for his fellow man and will build an enduring edifice of character within himself. The physician should ask of his destiny no more than this, and he should be content with no less."

Tinsley R. Harrison, MD
Author and Editor
Harrisons's *Principles of Internal Medicine*

During my medical training, I constantly sought out the great teachers. Their wagons were loaded. Associating with them, I surmised, was a wise thing to do. Dr. Tinsley Harrison had been the Professor and Chairman of the Department of Internal Medicine at The University Hospital in Birmingham. He was the author of the major medical textbook which was recognized around the world as "the bible" of medicine. After his retirement he moved to a nearby resort, Lake Martin, and taught a special clinical program at the Russell Hospital in Alexander City. The program allowed a medical student to study with him for a two-month period. I wish it could have been longer, but I discovered truth in an ancient Chinese proverb:

"A single conversation across the table with a wise man is worth a month's study of books."[1]

When I learned of this opportunity to study with a "giant" in the field of medicine, Susan and I packed our bags and Sted's toys and

---

[1]Chinese Proverb, *Motivational Quotes* p. 49.

went to Alexander City. (Chanee had not been born). We lived in a small, second-hand, two bedroom house trailer during that period. That didn't matter. I would have lived in a tent for the experience.

Dr. Harrison, the man, surpassed his reputation. He was a masterful diagnostician and often diagnosed complicated and rare diseases just by listening to a patient's medical history. To him, laboratory work and X-rays were used only to confirm his diagnosis. Although he was a human computer, he also possessed the rare characteristics of compassion and professionalism, which brought forth admiration from his patients and students alike. I found this common characteristic running through the veins of many great people I have known. It is a rare, but enviable trait.

To this day, when a patient is upset about his or her treatment, I can still hear Dr. Harrison say, "Never resent an affront offered by a sick man. The disturbed patient is often crying out for help. As physicians, it is our duty to help them through their crisis."

Dr. Harrison helped me through a difficult period in my professional development—a time when I was learning to think like a physician, not a football player. You know something, that's not an easy adjustment to make. He demonstrated to me and hundreds of others the standards by which physicians should honor their profession and treat their patients.

I was at a pivotal point in my life. It was time to bridge the gap which so many athletes face. Athletics had been a training ground, but being an athlete is not one's destiny. It is a temporary role in the game of life, and it's not easy to lay athletics aside. However, there comes a time in everyone's life when he must "hang it up." In the next chapter, we will look at how Coach Bryant wrestled with his decision and chose to retire as Alabama's football coach.

CHAPTER 13

COACH BRYANT MAKES THE DECISION

Alabama had lost only one game in Bryant-Denny Stadium in a quarter of a century. The University of Southern Mississippi and its great quarterback, Reggie Collier, were delivering the second to the 1982 Alabama team. I watched Coach Bryant closely on the sidelines as his team made one mistake after another, which ultimately cost Alabama the game. Something was terribly wrong. Ordinarily, he would be upset about the mistakes and penalties, pacing up and down the sidelines and reprimanding those who had committed foolish errors. That day, he stood there on the sidelines showing no external emotion. I knew there was a serious problem.

The next morning, Sunday, I went to the WBRC Television Studios in Birmingham where he did his weekly TV show. I felt the necessity to check on him.

He admitted that he had not slept all night. It showed. I asked if I could talk with him and he said "Yes, I need to talk to you." Following the television show, we went to lunch and I asked him what was wrong. He said "Gaylon, it is time for me to quit." "Coach," I said, "I have heard that you were going to get out of coaching every year since 1963. You can't quit now, just because things aren't going so well." "You don't understand", he said, "things are different now."

In 1971, he had turned the program around for a second time following two or three disappointing seasons. At that time, he was 12 years younger and in much better health. His health was the problem now and he knew it. Two years previously, he had had a stroke, but that fact had been kept from the media. Fortunately, he recovered, but was taking a number of medications to help control his cardio-vascular problems. Although he was one of the toughest, strong-willed individuals I have known, time had taken its toll. Few others could have gone as long as he had under the pressure and with similar medical problems.

He always said that when he felt that he was no longer able to do his job as *he* expected it to be done, he would step down. After explaining his situation to me that day, I understood and agreed that the decision he had made was the correct one. He loved his University and its athletic program too much to see it slide backward.

He said: "There are tough years ahead, because in the last three or four years, I have been ineffective as a recruiter. We are going to have to get someone in here who is young enough and tough enough to weather the storm that lies ahead. Alabama is in for some lean years, and our alumni won't understand why." He asked me to keep his retirement decision confidential. He had not yet talked with the president of the University of Alabama, Dr. Joab Thomas.

That same afternoon, he and the team accepted the bid to play in The Liberty Bowl against The University of Illinois. He knew then that it would be his last game as a coach. The team did not yet know about his decision.

Thanks to Ellis Taylor

Although I had played for him from 1961 through 1964, I never knew Paul W. Bryant, the individual, until many years later. He was my coach and my teacher. I had respected and feared him, but was in awe of the man and somewhat uncomfortable in his presence. He seemed to intimidate almost everyone else, too.

I owe the opportunity to have known him later as a friend and confidant to my good friend, Ellis Taylor, from Jasper, Alabama. Ellis is a great sportsman. He was one of the charter directors of the Alabama Sports Hall of Fame. Although he did not attend college there, he has been an important figure in the athletic programs at The University of Alabama. He and Coach Bryant had become close friends.

At the George Lindsey Celebrity Golf Tournament for the Alabama Special Olympics in Montgomery, Ellis recognized that I was somewhat uncomfortable around Coach, so he set out to correct that. He invited me to play golf with the two of them and Dale Robertson, the actor from Oklahoma. Ellis usually saw to it that Coach and I rode in the same golf cart. Slowly, the ice was broken.

Each summer, Ellis Taylor, Red Pope of Birmingham and several others, took the Alabama coaching staff to Florida to play golf and fish for four days. Following that weekend in Montgomery, Ellis invited me to come along with the Alabama group each year, and saw to it that Coach and I always played in the same foursome. Slowly, our friendship matured and Coach Bryant began to confide in me some of his medical and personal problems.

That new relationship is one I shall always treasure. I got to know the personal side of Coach Paul Bryant. He worried about the players who had quit football because he had gotten on their cases too hard. He felt that had he been a "little more patient," he could have kept each one and helped him grow as a player and as a person. He took

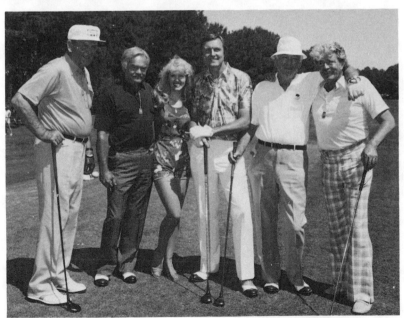

Coach Paul Bryant, Don Drummond, Gaylon McCollough, Ellis Taylor, and Dale Robertson with the tournament queen at the George Lindsey Golf Tournament in Montgomery, Alabama.

great pride in those who had gone through the entire football and educational program, but took it as a personal loss that he had "lost" so many others.

Coach Bryant was a religious man who wanted to do what was right and worried that he might not have lived the kind of life necessary to get him into heaven. I'm sure he is there. One only needed to see him with a child to see his kindness and how he melted in their hands. He became an inspiration to Chanee, our daughter, in her ice skating, because he gave her encouragement. She drew strength from him. His interest was genuine.

He chose to give his time and a great deal of money to young people so that many of them could have a better chance in life.

One of his last gifts to his former players was to establish a scholarship program for the sons and daughters of those who needed assistance in order for them to attend college.

Coach Bryant donated the first $100,000 towards the establishment of a Hall of Honor designed to pay tribute to all the players and coaches to whom he gave the credit for the 323 wins. That Hall of

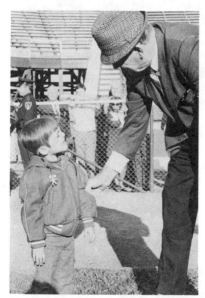

Coach Paul Bryant talks with Sted McCollough prior to the 1967 Alabama-Tennessee game.

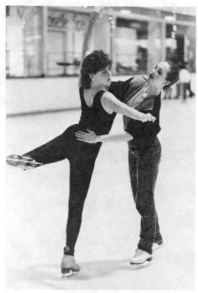

Chanee McCollough received a tip from one of the Russian skating coaches prior to the 1986 Goodwill games.

Honor will become a reality by 1987 in the new Bryant Center Complex on the campus of the University of Alabama.

One Christmas morning, he left his home in Tuscaloosa and drove to Birmingham to visit a sick child whose Christmas wish was to meet Coach Bryant. The stories about his generosity are endless. He did all these things not for show or public recognition, but because he was a good man and gained a great deal of pleasure from helping other people help themselves. He took, but he gave much, much more.

To my friend, Ellis Taylor, I shall always be grateful. He has opened many doors for me. A master at inter-personal relationships, he knew exactly what he was doing when he made it possible for me to know a side of Coach that few others have. I only wish I could have shared more time with Coach Bryant. There was so much to be learned. Fortunately, I am still loading my wagon with wisdom gained from his good friend, and mine, Ellis Taylor.

Selecting a New Coach

After the 1981 football season, Dr. Thomas reluctantly accepted Coach Bryant's resignation. A few weeks later, Dr. Thomas appointed a five-man selection committee for the purpose of choosing a new coach. The committee was composed of Dr. Thomas, as the chairman, Red Blount, Earnest Williams, Charles Scott and me. Mr. Blount, a Montgomery businessman, was also a former postmaster general of the United States, and a member of the University's Board of Trustees. Mr. Williams, another Trustee, had served on the selection committee which hired Coach Bryant in late 1957. Charlie Scott was chairman of a faculty athletic committee and an executive of the NCAA.

Before coming back to Alabama, Dr. Thomas had chosen a coach at North Carolina State using this same type of committee structure.

Initially, we were going to choose a "Head Coach Designate," a man who would come in and work for a year under Coach Bryant as did Tom Osborne at Nebraska before he took over for Bob Devaney. Coach Bryant had given Dr. Thomas a list of about twelve (12) qualified prospects for the job and asked that he have nothing else to with the selection. He felt that there were too many of his к players and coaches who would feel hurt if he had any more to do with the selection process. Coach asked me specifically to make sure that the record was straight on this issue.

For Coach Bryant, those were truly days of internal conflict. He wrestled with his decision. Should he stay on for another year as planned? Should he resign as the head coach and stay on as the athletic director, or should he resign completely? His decision to retire was one of the most significant sports stories of the decade. He was an institution—he knew the significance of what was to follow and recognized that the course of sports history in the state of Alabama was hanging in the balance. From day to day he vacillated. Dr. Thomas and I "twisted his arm" into staying on as the Athletic Director and agreed with him that, under the circumstances, hiring a head coach designate was a bad idea.

We were able to keep his retirement plans quiet until after the regular season was over. Then, Dr. Thomas contacted six of the twelve candidates given to him by Coach Bryant.

I remember the Thursday morning that I called Ray Perkins in New York to see if he would have any interest in the Alabama job. I was somewhat hesitant to pose the question to Ray, because one would think that when a man who wants to be a football coach becomes the head coach of the New York Giants he has ascended to the pinnacle of the profession. "Ray," I said, "Coach Bryant has decided to retire. On Sunday the selection committee plans to interview some people to take the job. Would you have any interest in talking to Dr. Thomas about it?"

In the typical Ray Perkins style, there was absolute silence on the other end of the phone lines for about 10 seconds. Then he responded in a confident, business-like voice, without reservation, "You're damn right I am."

I admit, at the time, I was shocked at his direct, no wishy-washy response, but that's how Ray Perkins is. There was no beating around the bush. I should have remembered that from our playing days. The same morning Dr. Thomas contacted him and his name was added to the list of prospective new head coaches.

The committee met on a Sunday in mid-December and interviewed the seven. Four candidates were interviewed in Tuscaloosa in Dr. Thomas' office on the campus. The three others were interviewed in my office in Birmingham. It was somewhat of a juggling act to schedule the interviews so that no candidate knew that the others were there. Miraculously, however, we managed to do so.

When the seven had been interviewed, there was no question as to who should be chosen. It quickly became obvious that Ray Perkins had the right background, skills, and intelligence to do the job, but equally as important, his steel blue eyes told everyone on the committee that he wanted the job. It had been a life-long ambition that he had never before divulged. The committee's decision was unanimous. It must have been Ray Perkins' destiny to become Alabama's head coach.

Coach Bryant had told us that the University's football program would need someone who was young and tough to weather the stormy days to follow. The committee felt that it needed a man who loved the University of Alabama over all others and who wanted, more than anything else, to be the person to carry on the tradition which had been built by the great coaches of the past.

When all was said and done, it was clear that Ray Perkins possessed all of the necessary requirements that Coach Bryant and Dr. Thomas had expected from the next head coach. Frankly, we did not think that we could hire him from the New York Giants to come back to a college job. The opportunity was offered to him, and he accepted. All knew, including Ray himself, that he would be subjected to much criticism and second guessing as he came back "home" to establish his own program at the University. He had been tested by the New York press and knew how to handle criticism.

Ray Perkins accepted a nearly impossible challenge, but anyone who knows him also remembers that he has never backed down from hard work or insurmountable odds.

When Coach Bryant was notified of the committee's choice, he was very pleased and immediately pledged his full support to helping Ray establish his own program. He also pledged to step down from the Athletic Director's position if he felt that his continued presence was interfering with Ray's program.

Alabama had a new coach, the best man for the job. He would need time and the support of all loyal Alabama people to build the program back, because he was certainly going to be subjected to tremendous scrutiny. At least, in the beginning, he would not have the full support of ALL Alabama fans.

In those days two groups of people followed and supported Alabama football. There are those who love the University and what it stands for—they are *true* Alabama Fans. Then there was a group who were fans of Coach Bryant, the man. Some people certainly fell into both categories. Those who were only Coach Bryant fans would never have been satisfied regardless of who was selected to be the next coach. There may never be another like him. I believe that Ray Perkins would be the first to admit that. Ray has often said that he was not at Alabama to *replace* Coach Bryant, but that he was honored to be the coach who followed him.

S.D. Gordon once said, "Shoes divide men into three classes. Some men wear their father's shoes, they make no decisions of their own. Some are unthinkingly shod (controlled) by the crowd. The strong man is his own cobbler, he insists on making his own choices. He walks in his own shoes."

Perkins is definitely not afraid of "making his own choices." He had a job to do. He and Coach Bryant knew what needed to be done.

Ray Perkins knows about "giants." He has been associated with a few in his days. He accepted his new challenge from the shoulders of the New York Giants, and two of his former coaches (Don Shula and Coach Bryant) are each giants. History will record that he was the man who best fit the bill to become the next in the series.

Coach Bryant had a right to be pleased when he learned the committee's choice. He knew the future of Alabama athletics was in good hands. Another former Alabama end had heard "Mama call" and came home—a destiny of choice, his and the selection committee's.

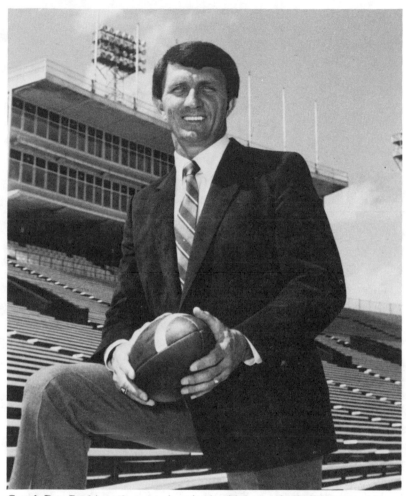

Coach Ray Perkins, the next giant in the Alabama football legacy.

CHAPTER 14

THE TORCH IS PASSED

Three days after the selection committee made its decision, a two way press conference was held between Tuscaloosa and New York City. Until the phone hook-ups were made between the two cities, only the members of the selection committee, Coach Bryant, and Ray Perkins, knew about the decisions of the past week. Dr. Thomas had done an excellent job in handling a delicate situation and keeping it from the press, who certainly would have tried to decide among themselves who should be selected. Such an unfortunate event would have divided Alabama people into many camps.

Before Coach Bryant made his statement of resignation to the press, the two of us sat in his office discussing the future. There seemed to be no regret and no remorse. He said the time had come. He had made the choice to "hang it up." He felt good about what had been done and was looking forward to having the opportunity to do some things he had always wanted to do. Primarily, he was concerned about some obstacles Ray Perkins would face as the new coach and was looking forward to helping him. But he quickly added, "When I feel I am getting in his way, I am going to get out altogether. I will never interfere."

Following some arm-twisting, he had agreed to teach a course in the regular college curriculum. Several years previously he had deservedly been given an honorary Ph.D. by the University. The subject matter for the new course would include organizational, motivational and management techniques one needs to deal with the problems in the real world—the same type of things he had taught so many of his players. He had agreed to stay on and share his philosophy of achievement with all students at the University who could register for his class. Because he loved the University of Alabama, he wanted to continue to contribute in every way he could.

He was hoping that his new college course might encourage some "walk-ons" to come to Alabama and might help some of those riding the fence to decide to come there, even if he wasn't coaching. He wanted so much for Ray Perkins to be successful and was looking forward to working with him.

Piercing Accusations

Coach Bryant came by our home to visit Susan and me on Monday night before he was hospitalized the next evening for chest pains. His greatest concerns that night were about the recruiting wars and some cruel accusations which had been made about him and against Ray Perkins by competitors. He was deeply hurt. This problem weighed heavily upon him. It showed in his face and eyes and I believe had a direct effect upon what happened thirty-six hours later. As he left, Susan said to me, "Coach doesn't look good." "Sue," I said, "he looks about the same to me tonight as he has for the past month." "Something's different tonight," she added. Maybe women do have a special intuition. I'm a doctor. I should have picked up on it myself, but I didn't. Looking back, I think he knew his time was running short. He had not been well for months.

"Time Just Ran Out"

A day and a half later, I was sitting in the conference room of my Clinic talking with a representative of the University, John Blackburn. He had come up to see me about serving on a committee to help build the Hall of Honor within the new Bryant Center Complex on the campus. This project was conceived by Coach Bryant to honor all the players and coaches who contributed to the 323 victories. At that same moment in a Tuscaloosa hospital, Coach Bryant had a massive heart attack and died suddenly. I believe if he had a choice, he would have wanted to go quickly. Dr. Tinsley Harrison once said, "A man who lives with dignity should be allowed to die with dignity." Coach Bryant experienced both.

The news of his death shocked the country. America had lost a hero, a legend, a giant upon whose shoulders so many had climbed in order to improve their chances to succeed. Alabama had lost a man who had brought more honor and prestige to the state than any other single human being in its history. His death left a void in the hearts and minds of all who knew him, or even knew of him.

Rarely does anyone pass through this world whose life affects the way large numbers of people think and behave. Many of us had the good fortune to know a man who did. His true greatness did not lie in the records his teams established nor in the individual accomplishments of the athletes who played for him. Coach Bryant quietly and surely established his place in history through his lasting effect upon all of those individuals whose lives he touched. He was sensitive, honest, fair, dedicated, loyal and unselfish, giving all credit for success to others and voluntarily taking the blame when things went awry.

Seeing people achieve more than they thought they could gave him great satisfaction. He never caved in following defeat, and never allowed us to do so either. "Hold your heads up high and walk with pride," he said, "You have class, show it. You were never beaten, time just ran out on you."

On January 26, 1983, time just ran out on him. Although he had done everything any human needed to do, he had not done several things he wanted to do.

Now, those of us who loved him must carry on with his unfinished business, supporting *his* University and its football tradition. I know that is how he would have willed it to us, his football family.

"Thanks for the Memories"

The tribute paid to him on the day of his burial was one befitting a king. As the procession passed Bryant-Denny Stadium and the practice field where his empty tower stood, it was almost more than one could bear. It seemed too final to think that this would be the last time he would pass by the areas where he had spent much of his professional life and where millions had paid tribute to him and his teams.

It is estimated that more than 300,000 people lined the road between Tuscaloosa and Birmingham to honor him as he passed by. Signs saying, "Thanks for the memories" and "We love you, Bear," proclaimed the respect and love Alabama fans had for their hero.

It was interesting to see the contrasts between generations. Those who looked old enough to have experienced World Wars I and II stood at attention and saluted as his procession passed, while most people of today's generation stood or sat reverently, but casually, as they watched the procession enroute to Elmwood Cemetery in Birmingham.

In Good Hands

He was gone, but his memory would live on in the minds and hearts of Americans forever. His life will serve as a beacon for everyone who respects pride, dignity, class and the work ethic. He was a role model for each of us to attempt to emulate. All who were touched by him are better people for having had the opportunity to know him. A legend was established and passed along. Now the responsibility lies on the shoulders of his students, our generation.

A few weeks later, Dr. Thomas appointed Ray Perkins Athletic Director. The tradition established by the giants of the past is safe. Joey Jones in his new book said that the future of the football program at Alabama is "In Good Hands."

Ray Perkins is young and tough. He has weathered the storm that Coach Bryant predicted was sure to come. It did. It appears to have passed, but all will not be smooth sailing—not in the game of football, nor in the game of life.

CHAPTER 15

"ALABAMA IS BACK"

On December 1, 1985, in what has come to be declared THE most exciting game of the series, Ray Perkins' Alabama team beat a fine Auburn team 25-23 and he declared "Alabama is back."

In the *Birmingham News* on the following Monday, Charles Hollis agreed. He wrote,

> "Once upon a time in the Land of Legends—before Ray Perkins succeeded one by the name of Paul W. Bryant - thousands and thousands of Alabama fans took their football for granted.
>
> They took:
>   Winning for granted.
>   Going to bowls for granted.
>   Making first downs for granted.
>
> If you were an outsider two or three years ago, and watching your first Alabama game in person, more than likely you would have been disappointed at what you saw.
>
> Everywhere you turned you would have seen spectators just sitting there, their arms folded, their legs crossed, yet seldom expressing any serious emotion.

If someone intercepted a pass, or scored a touchdown, or did anything that might be defined as a big play, most of the Alabama spectators would not move.

Instead of jumping out of their seats, they just sat there, with their arms folded, with their legs crossed, and clapping three or four times.

Not even a loud clap, either.

You would have sworn you were attending the ballet or a golf match instead of an Alabama football game.

That's what winning will do.

That's what taking success for granted will do.

In Alabama's case, with Coach Bryant producing six national championships and 13 SEC titles over a quarter of a century, there was a whole lot to be spoiled about.

Then one day Bryant was gone, and . . . Perkins . . . was on the block.

At first things went well.

When Perkins went 8-4 his first year, including a 28-7 upset of SMU in the Sun Bowl, The Alabama family began to reach and accept him. (I think he should have been named "Coach of the Year" in the SEC for the job he did that year).

Then his second team dropped to 5-6 for the school's worst season in 27 years (the storm Coach Bryant had predicted) and, suddenly, some of the fans who had welcomed him into the UA (University of Alabama) family the year before, were now wondering if he was the right man to replace a legend.

Fortunately, for Perkins, though, the Crimson Tide upended Auburn 17-15 in the final game of the season.

Out of the darkness of a 5-6 season, however, came a re-birth of Alabama football and a new brand of Crimson Tide religion more intense than ever.

Where once the crowds were rather passive, now they were getting carried away by their team.

For the first time in years Alabama fans appear to be as hungry for winning as the football team was after going 5-6 in 1984.

And when the Tide rebounded with an 8-2-1 record this season including Saturday's 25-23 victory over Auburn, Perkins proclaimed to his players afterward: 'Alabama is back!'

Time will answer that. (I think the verdict is already in).

But by beating Auburn for the second straight year—for the second straight year when his team was the under-dog—Perkins has taken a giant step in that direction. Once again the Crimson Tide is ruling the state—the way it did in the '60s and '70s.

Perkins has said that he is one recruiting class away from having his program back to competing for the national title on a regular basis. (Forrest Davis, one of the south's lead-ing recruiting analysts, reported on 2/12/86 that Alabama has just signed the best group of high school athletes in its history, maybe the best in the nation).

Alabama signed 15 players from what is generally consid-ered to be the top 30 or so in the South.

And to entice future recruits, Perkins is talking with Uni-versity of Hawaii officials about adding a 12th game to Ala-bama's schedule, possibly within the next three years.

The Aloha Bowl in Honolulu was Bama's bowl in 1985. It drew the ire of many Alabama fans and alumni because of the inconvenience and cost to get there. Even band mem-bers criticized Perkins for accepting an Aloha invitation.

'I think it's wrong for our fans and alumni to criticize Coach Perkins,' said offensive guard David Gilmer. 'What a lot of people don't realize, is that it was the seniors who voted to go to the Aloha. We really had the final say—not like some coaches do with their seniors.'

'Considering the options Alabama had—Cherry, Holiday, Bluebonnet and Liberty—the seniors felt it was best to go to the Aloha,' Gilmer added. 'I know we won't have a lot of fans there, but a bowl is supposed to be a reward at the end of the season, and no one knows how hard we've worked to have the kind of season our fans can be proud of.

'Nothing in the world would make me feel better than to have my mother and little brother in Hawaii over Christmas to watch me play. But like I told mom the other day . . . she wasn't out there during three-a-days (for two weeks in August) and doing all the sweating and hurting.

"No one wanted to help bring Alabama back this year more than Coach Perkins and the players. When a lot of people gave up on us, and a lot of people did, and really criticized Coach Perkins for the kind of job he was doing, he stood behind us and never gave up on us.

'When you think about what Coach Perkins had done following a legend like Coach Bryant, I don't think there's another coach alive who could have done any better." (The selection committee thought so too, David).

Alabama beat the University of Southern California in the Aloha Bowl, 24—3, and ended the year with an overall record of 9-2-1, its best in several years.

Ray Perkins and Dr. Joab Thomas make a great leadership team. Both are men of integrity and purpose. They are also experts in their fields. Each wants what is best for *his* University. Together, they can work through the difficult problems which lie ahead.

At the 1986 meeting of the Southeastern Conference, the University of Alabama stood firm against easing penalties levied on schools sanctioned for rule violations. All other SEC presidents and athletic directors favored rescinding prior financial sanctions and rewarded wrong doing—interesting.

Given the time, the athletes, and the support they need, the Thomas-Perkins team will keep Alabama in its traditional place—at the top. Leaders need troops while the war is on, not when the battle has been won. Has anyone looked at the 1986 schedule? Alabama and its fans will be tested.

UNIVERSITY OF ALABAMA
1986 FOOTBALL SCHEDULE
Head Coach: Ray Perkins

Aug.	27	Ohio State (Kickoff Classic) (at E. Rutherford, N.J.)	8:00 EDT
SEPT.	**6**	**VANDERBILT†**	**1:30 CDT**
SEPT.	**13**	**SOUTHERN MISSISSIPPI‡**	**1:30 CDT**
Sept.	20	at Florida	1:30 EDT
OCT.	**4**	**NOTRE DAME‡**	**1:30 CDT**
OCT.	**11**	**MEMPHIS STATE† (HC)** . .	**1:30 CDT**
Oct.	18	at Tennessee	1:30 EDT
OCT.	**25**	**PENN STATE†**	**1:30 CDT**
NOV.	1	at Mississippi State	1:30 CST
NOV.	**8**	**LOUISIANA STATE‡**	**1:30 CST**
NOV.	**15**	**TEMPLE†**	**1:30 CST**
NOV.	**29**	**AUBURN‡**	**1:30 CST**

†at Tuscaloosa   ‡at Birmingham

PART III

A LOOK AT MEDICINE

CHAPTER 16

ARCHITECTURAL MEDICINE

"Do not wish to be anything but what you are and try to be that perfectly."[1]

With the foundation laid, it was time to get on with the training for my chosen career. Just as my parents had told me since childhood, education would be the key that would open the doors to success.

In 1968, while in medical school, I attended a lecture that shaped my professional career. A plastic surgeon on the hospital staff spoke to our class and presented an overview of the broad field of *general* plastic surgery. When I saw what could be done to faces, I knew at that moment that I had finally discovered the field of medicine for which I was suited. My professional destiny flashed before my eyes.

Case after case of patients whose faces had been altered by carefully planned and executed plastic surgical procedures were projected on the screen of the same lecture room where I had endured the necessary lectures on Pharmacology, Biochemistry and Preventive Medicine. Children who were deformed by birth defects were made to look "normal." Through reconstructive plastic surgery, men and women who had been disfigured by accidents and cancer were

---

[1]St. Frances DeSales, *Motivational Quotes* p. 33.

made whole again. Years of aging seemed to be brushed away by the surgeon's hands with cosmetic surgical procedures. People who lacked beauty or handsomeness emerged as attractive men and women by altering their noses, chins, and other features. Their self-images improved as dramatically as their appearances.

"This" I said to myself "is truly remarkable. It would be wonderful to be able to do those things for people. This is my destiny."

For the first time, the screen lit up with subject matter which seemed tailor made for me.

Since childhood, I had had an interest in both medicine and architecture. Plastic surgery, I concluded, is architectural medicine. I was so stimulated that I cut my next two classes and went straight to the medical school library. Pulling out the books on plastic surgery and examining before-and-after pictures, I realized that I had finally found my specialty in medicine, plastic surgery of the face.

Very early, I realized that the field of *general* plastic surgery was so all-encompassing that no one could master every aspect of it. I remembered what Dr. Porch told me several years previously in Miami: "We are entering an era of specialization." So, I decided to carve out one aspect of the field of plastic surgery, the face, and become the best I could be in that particular area.

Since I had been a small boy, I had enjoyed creating new things and drawing faces. For hours, I would sit and sketch, trying to duplicate the portraits of famous people, studying the details of eyes, noses and chins. The human face is intriguing because it represents the portion of each person's body which is truly unique.

Changing one's face can often change one's life. The eyes have been called the window to the soul; the configuration of the chin depicts masculinity or femininity; and the nose is the most prominent and most variable feature of the face.

Helen of Troy had the face that "launched a thousand ships." The faces of many of the great men and women of yesteryear, whose wisdom has endured through the ages, have been preserved by the masters.

Facts About Facial Plastic Surgery

In 1985, across the United States, more than two million people chose to undergo elective surgery for the sole purpose of improving their appearances. Many more had procedures designed to reconstruct a portion of the body following an accident, tumor surgery, or a congenital defect.

A recent national survey (*Psychology Today*) indicates that almost one-half of all Americans are dissatisfied with the shape of their noses and one out of four are dissatisfied with their "chins" (and necks). Furthermore, 25% of all cosmetic surgery is performed on men, and that percentage is increasing.

For what reason would a healthy individual ask to be subjected to surgery knowing that the possibility of potentially serious problems exists? The answer is to attempt to improve the QUALITY of their life.

Today's America is a youth-oriented society with a strong emphasis on appearance. It is common knowledge that the business community seeks attractive people to fill available positions. Those who have the responsibility of hiring new employees confirm that a pleasing appearance weighs heavily when all other qualifications are equal. Is it any wonder that many patients who have cosmetic plastic surgery do so for economic reasons? Not only is this true for the fashion model, television and movie personality, corporate executive or the professional person, but for anyone whose work requires that they interact with the public. Educators know that the young people they teach relate better to one who does not look old or poorly groomed.

The facts are that not only do people in the upper socio-economic bracket choose to undergo facial plastic surgery, but so do working people living on a budget. Most people plan for their cosmetic surgery just like they plan for a vacation, a new piece of jewelry, or an automobile. It is viewed as an investment in themselves.

When one looks better, his pride and ego are bolstered, and not so surprisingly, it has been shown that when he feels good about himself he performs better. Thank goodness for vanity. Without it no one would bathe, shave, care for their hair, coordinate their clothes, watch their weight, or care about the impression one makes on his fellow man. The cave man society was free of vanity. We are approaching the 21st century.

Madison Avenue advertising firms certainly understand the value Americans place upon personal appearance. Billions of dollars are spent each year by these "average Americans" on cosmetics, accessories, fashionable wardrobes, vitamins, health foods and weight

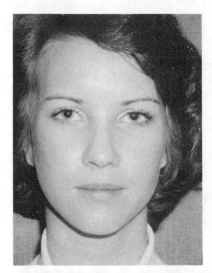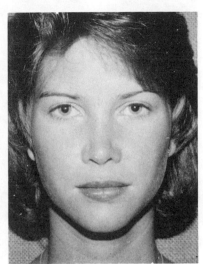

A wide nose can be improved by repositioning the nasal bones and cartilages and removing any excess.

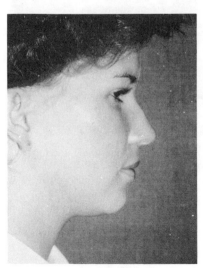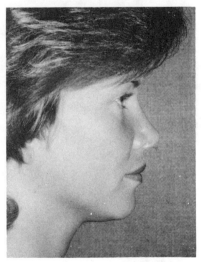

Supporting the nasal tip and removal of a bony and cartilagenous hump can often produce dramatic improvement in one's appearance and bolster self-esteem.

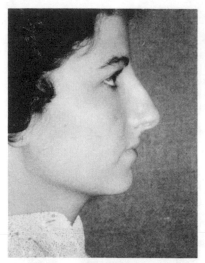 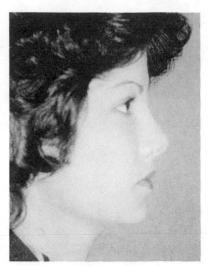

A nose that is too large is "out of proportion" to the other facial features. Reducing its size and altering its shape brings it into harmony and enhances the other facial features. (A direct brow lift was also performed to correct her sagging brows.)

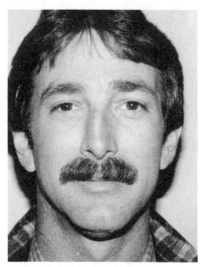 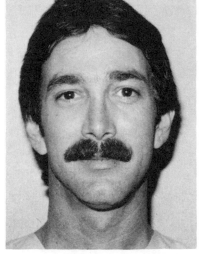

A crooked nose may result from an injury, previously unsuccessful surgery or may be a family trait. When associated with internal deformities, such as a deviated nasal septum, the patient may experience breathing difficulties. A functional nasal plastic operation can often improve both the appearance and airway.

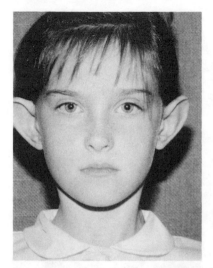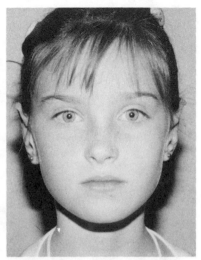

Large or protruding ears can be repositioned with the otoplasty procedure. Although the size of the ears are not changed, they assume a much more natural relationship to the head.

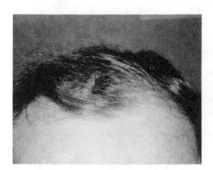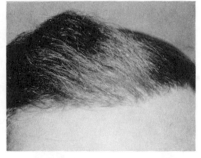

The best time to begin hair transplantation is when the frontal hairline begins to recede. Hair transplantation can camouflage additional hair loss.

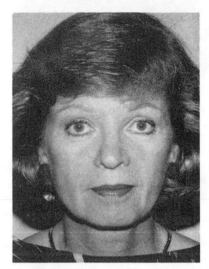 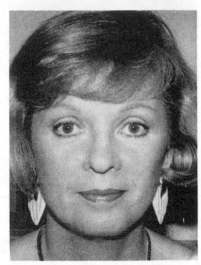

Early correction of the signs of aging is demonstrated in this woman after upper and lower eyelid surgery, a forehead, cheek-neck lift, and submental lipectomy.

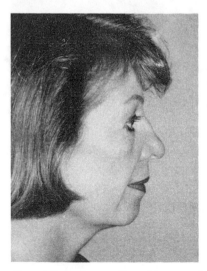 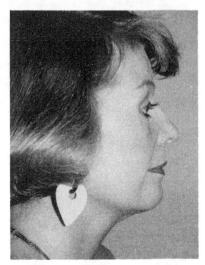

Correction of a receding chin can add the finishing touch.

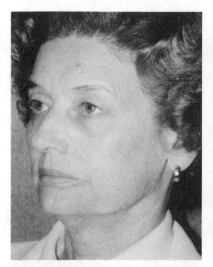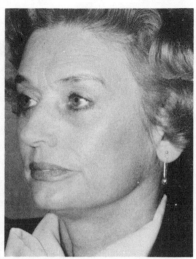

*This woman underwent a face lift, upper and lower lid blepharoplasty and
a chemical peel around her lips. Surgery helps correct sags and bulges,
peeling is necessary for wrinkles.*

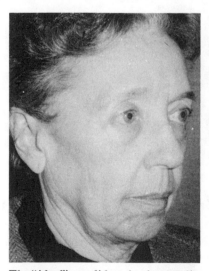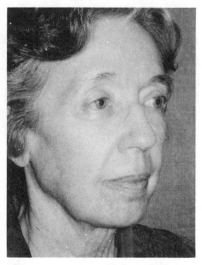

*The "ideal" candidate for face peeling—deep creases around the mouth
and eyes plus the weather-damaged appearance of the rest of the facial skin
result from years of sun and wind exposure. The chemical peel can often
give the skin a much more youthful and "fresher" appearance. No surgery,
other than the peel, was performed.*

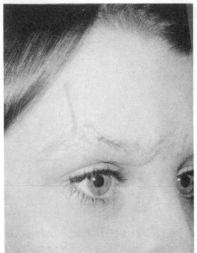

Figure A

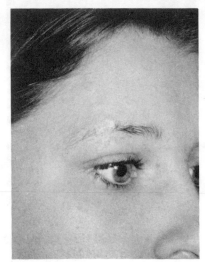

Figure B

Dermabrasion is an invaluable component of scar revision surgery. The scars depicted in this patient required two stages. The scar was first excised and closed with a zig-zag plasty (geometric broken line). (figure B)

Six months later the elevated edges were dermabraded, or sanded down, leaving a much smoother contour.

Figure C represents the final result six months after the dermabrasion.

The dermabrasion procedure was performed with a rotating wire brush under local anesthesia.

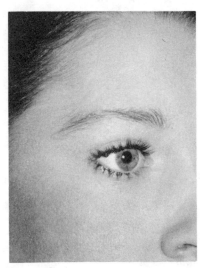

Figure C

control products. These are the same individuals who choose to have facial plastic surgery.

Cosmetic (or aesthetic) plastic surgery can often improve one's appearance by correction of deformed or unsightly facial features and by eliminating some of the conspicuous marks of the aging process.

Reconstructive plastic surgery is that which attempts to restore portions of the face, nose, head, and neck to the state which might have existed prior to an injury, infection, tumor removal, or previously unsuccessful surgery. Correction of many congenital defects also fall under this category.

Much has been written in the lay press about cosmetic plastic surgery. Unfortunately, the information is generally presented by the writer to be a "grabber" or to promote one group of surgeons over another as part of a coordinated expensive advertising campaign. Because of this, the public has many misconceptions about this field. In the pages to follow, I will attempt to put the surgery and those who perform it in perspective—now that I have become part of the system.

Why Be A Specialist?

"Specialization is always a matter of subtraction from a well balanced whole."[2]

Specialization is the process by which all professions learn more about any subject. After a thorough examination of *facial* plastic surgery, the parts to the puzzle fell into place—architecture, art and medicine, the perfect merger. I would be a specialist in Surgery of the Face. The other aspects of *general* plastic surgery—burns, hand surgery, cancer reconstruction, bed sores, breast surgery and body contouring—never really appealed to me. Since I did not intend to do any of those types of surgery, I didn't see the purpose of spending valuable time pursuing something I didn't want or need. I needed to focus my energies on the main target, my destiny of choice.

---

[2]Thomas F. Heinze, *Creation vs. Evolution Handbook* (The Baker Book House, 1973), p. 97.

CHAPTER 17

TO BE A FACIAL SURGEON

The more I learned about the sub-specialty of "*facial* plastic surgery," the more certain I was of my career choice. It was the logical option for a young surgeon who also had an interest in architecture. With the final objective in focus, the journey began. I began to plan my career as a facial surgeon.

Board Certification

After a great deal of research, I discovered that there were two routes to achieve my goal and become a *board-certified* surgeon—one direct and one more circuitous. The direct route could take me through an accredited residency program in head and neck surgery (ENT) to become board-certified. Using this approach, I would spend all four years working on the face and in the head and neck region. What better way to learn the anatomy and physiology of the face and surrounding structures? In addition to the residency, I could complete a year of specialized training (a fellowship) in plastic surgery of the face. That certainly would be the most direct route and provide the maximum training in the face, head and neck during that five-year period.

There was another possible route, however. The staff plastic surgeon at the University Hospital in Birmingham explained that it would also be possible to complete a four year general surgery residency and then take a two or three year residency in general plastic surgery to become a practitioner of general plastic surgery. During the general surgery residency, however, the amount of surgical experience and direct training in the face would be extremely limited and there would be essentially *no* training in surgery of the nose, chin, ears and eyelids. During the two year *general* plastic surgery residency, it would be necessary to study burn surgery, hand surgery, cancer surgery, correction of congenital defects and all the other plastic procedures over the body. In order to become board-certified by the general plastic surgery board, I surmised, a relatively small amount of time would be spent refining my skills in plastic surgery of the face and nose, which is what I wanted. I talked with a number of other people whose opinions I respected and all of them advised me to go the direct route. Their reason had merit. Become a specialist.

After examining my options, the choice seemed rather simple. If I had decided to take a trip from Birmingham to New York (assuming New York was my goal), I could go directly there or could go first to Miami, then Houston, then San Diego, then San Francisco, then to Chicago and then on to New York. I wasn't interested in taking a tour through the broad field of surgery. When we can finally put things in perspective and cut through all the "bull", the logical decisions become simple. Most things seem difficult until the answer is revealed. I quickly realized that the more direct route not only allowed me to get to my goal quicker and more efficiently, but provided even more detailed training and surgical experience in the specific region of the body, the face, in which I intended to spend the rest of my professional career.

This decision was not unlike the choice I made between the University of Alabama and Georgia Tech. It was made with thoughtful consideration knowing that there would be hurdles to overcome. Some people would think I should have made another choice. It is impossible to please everyone, so we have to please ourselves and do what we think is right for us, even though it may go against public opinion.

The Shoe That Fits

Later, I discovered that some other surgeons who had chosen to practice general plastic surgery would take serious offense to the basic facts about there being *two* educational routes to the same destination. Maybe this was because they hadn't investigated their alternatives prior to making their own choices. I guess each person has to justify his own decisions in life.

> *"The shoe that fits one person pinches another; there is no recipe for living that suits all cases. . ."*[1]

The shoe fit my foot. I decided to wear it.

Pinching Some Toes

Now that I had a game plan, it would become important to see that the parts of the puzzle fit. I quickly realized that there would be obstacles to overcome and people who would attempt to stand in my way. My new plan might be viewed as a threat and pinch some toes—like going to Alabama in pursuit of a national championship ring. It became important to identify the obstacles and put together a team that could help me achieve my goal, as I had seen done throughout my athletic career.

The director of the Division of Otolaryngology (ENT or head and neck surgery) at the University of Alabama Hospitals and Clinics was Dr. James J. Hicks. He and his brother, Dr. Julius N. Hicks, grew up in Enterprise, too. They had been instrumental in helping me get accepted to medical school. I talked with them about my plan to become a facial surgeon and they agreed to help once more.

My residency training program to become board-certified in otolaryngology (head and neck surgery) was set to begin some two years down the road. In the meantime, I set out to get as much training as possible with the staff surgeons at the University Hospital and with the private practitioners of plastic and reconstructive surgery in Birmingham.

---

[1] Carl Jung, *Bartlett's Quotations.*

The Changing Face of Medicine

Things went exactly as planned during the period preceding my residency. My internship with the Baptist Hospitals was both educational and enlightening. During that time, I had an opportunity to meet many doctors and surgeons who were already in private practice around the various regions of Birmingham. I saw how many of them dealt with each other, with organized medicine, and with their patients. In that group of doctors there were some outstanding men and women. On the other hand, there were some disappointments. I quickly learned that doctors are only human beings who have gone to school longer. Physicians are part of the medical team trying to win the battle for good health and well-being. The M.D. carries with it a responsibility to mankind and to fellow physicians.

Hippocrates, the great physician, established the oath of integrity. Each physician took the Hippocratic oath on the day he or she was awarded a degree from medical school. I later found out that the same "oath" could have many different meanings depending upon who was interpreting it.

Upon graduation, each physician is given the same chance. The human element determines how each will use the degree to best serve his profession, his specialty, his fellow man and himself. Some would climb upon giant shoulders in order to achieve greater heights; some would just observe, others would complain and do nothing, like many of the athletes I had encountered. Some of the physicians whose paths I crossed were giants upon whose shoulders the future of medicine would rest.

A Competitive Business

During my internship, I realized that the practice of medicine is a competitive business containing the elements of jealousy, politics, and ruthlessness. It was a rude awakening.

Someone always seems to be throwing up a defense to keep us from reaching our goal. The decision one makes in responding to a given situation is dependent upon genetic and environmental factors.

The story is told of a man who had two sons, one a pessimist, the other an optimist. When put into a store full of toys the pessimistic son did not play with a single one for fear of breaking them all. When put into a barn full of horse manure, the optimistic son immediately sprang into action proclaiming, "with all this manure, there has to be a pony in here somewhere!"

As corporations, hospitals, government, and medical fraternity groups scramble to control where patients may go for health care, doctors tend to lose their allegiance to their profession, and, therefore, professionalism yields to commercialism. Without being pessimistic, the fact is that the "oneness" (Coach Bryant's concept of teamwork) that has existed among physicians is slowly, but surely, beginning to disintegrate—a process of premeditated erosion.

What do you think happens in those corporate board meetings? Corporations look upon physicians as the key in obtaining control of patient flow. Corporate charters are not based upon the ethics described by Hippocrates. The health care magnates of The New York Stock Exchange seem to be gaining control of the medical profession, dictating what doctors and health institutions do. Private or local medical institutions are being acquired by larger conglomerates whose primary objective seems to be to elevate the price of their stock on Wall Street and gobble up everything in their paths. The physician staff and ultimately the patients become a commodity which can be traded to the highest (or lowest) bidder. The public should pay closer attention to what happens on Wall Street or on Capitol Hill. One stroke of legislation can abolish a hundred years of tradition.

During this commercialization process, many doctors are becoming employees of health care corporations, believing that they have no other choice. A recent AMA survey concluded that approximately 60% of licensed physicians in the United States are already under some kind of contractural agreement with a hospital, federal agency, or corporate conglomerate. Like that of the professional athlete, the physician professional's contract will become a commodity subjected to the skills of the negotiators of the conglomerate team.

Unless challenged, slowly, but surely, socialization and commercialization of the delivery of medicine will interfere with freedom of choice. The patient will be directed to a particular institution or group of physicians that has a contractural arrangement with whomever pays for their medical care or insurance premiums. As a consumer, I want to choose which hospital or clinic I go to for my health care and select the physician in whose hands I put my life. As a physician, I would prefer to care for those patients who come to me because they have chosen to do so.

An Independent Clinic

Seeing the trend toward "centralization of health services" some 12 years ago, I sought an alternative for my patients. My plan to establish an independent out-patient surgical clinic for the delivery of facial plastic surgical services would cut the high costs of hospital based surgery, allow freedom of choice, and preserve patient privacy. I was convinced that the concept had validity and I set out to make the dream a reality.

> *"Some men see things as they are and say 'Why?'"*
> *"I dream things that never were, and say "Why not?"*[2]

A New Era

Some eleven years later, in the December 15, 1985 edition of *PARADE*, Donald Robinson explained that "We Can Stay Healthy For

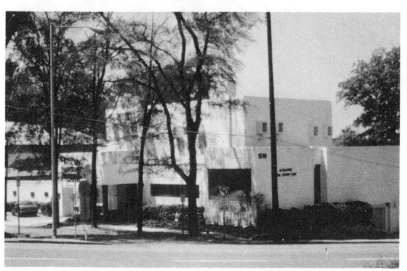

The McCollough Facial Surgery Clinic near the UAB Medical Center complex.

[2]George Bernard Shaw, *Motivational Quotes* p. 25.

Less" by taking advantage of the changes in health care. He explained that there is a "revolution taking place in the way Americans receive health care." One of the changes is a shift toward outpatient surgery. Some insurance companies even pay extra whenever surgery is performed on an outpatient basis. The president of the national Blue Cross and Blue Shield Association was quoted as saying, "We want to encourage physicians to keep patients out of the hospital."

The evolutionary process has taken years to develop, and I might say faced great resistance, as we shall soon see.

CHAPTER 18

THREE GIANTS ...
ONE AMERICA

"Because it is common sense doesn't mean it is common practice."[1]

Once the choice had been made to become a facial surgeon and establish my clinic, the first thing I had to do was to obtain the training necessary to perform the type of surgery I intended to do. Almost miraculously, things began to fall in place.

During residency training, each of our residents was allowed to attend one national medical convention. When my turn came, I had a choice between Houston and Tampa. Although I had almost become a Dallas Cowboy, I had never been to the state of Texas. Houston was my choice. I now realize that it was definitely the right choice.

As I went about researching careers in plastic surgery, I heard about a surgeon in New Orleans whose practice was limited to plastic surgery of the face. His was the type of practice that I had hoped to develop, therefore, I had planned to contact him at the appropriate time for advice and direction.

When I walked into the large meeting room at Houston's Galleria Hotel, a surgeon was lecturing about making chins larger in order to

---

[1]Anonymous, *Friends* (Kaplans).

enhance the appearance of one's face. Marilyn Monroe's picture was up on a screen. He said, "This is one of the most famous people known to have had a chin implant." I moved to the front row and tried to digest every word. This was the man I needed to meet, Dr. Jack Anderson, the facial plastic surgeon from New Orleans. What a coincidence! (Was it a coincidence or destiny? Maybe my plan would materialize sooner than I thought.)

The next morning Ed Stevenson, an ENT-Head and Neck Surgeon from Birmingham, introduced me to him and I told Dr. Anderson about my dream. When he agreed to help, I was on my way. He allowed me to visit New Orleans to watch him work for a month. During that month, Susan, Sted, Chanee and I moved into a small student apartment in the Tulane Medical Center. Dr. Anderson later helped me set up my facial plastic fellowship training through The American Academy of Facial Plastic and Reconstructive Surgery, Inc. He is one of the founders and presidents of that organization. Today, it is the largest organization of specialty plastic surgeons in the world.

The Fellowship

The next year would prove to be an intensive study program from morning to late afternoon at the side of three giants in *"general"* and *"specialty"* plastic surgery—Dr. Jack Anderson in New Orleans, Dr. Walter Berman in Beverly Hills, and Dr. Richard Webster in Boston. Each had been selected because of his expertise in the field and because of his teaching abilities. My family not only had the most enlightening educational experience of our lives, but a wonderful opportunity to live in three distinctive areas of The United States.

Anderson

"When the storm clouds come in, the eagles soar while the small birds take cover."[2]

In Yiddish, there is a word, "chutzpah," which means "incredible

---

[2]*Ibid*

guts." Leaders must have chutzpah. Jack Anderson does. In order to effectively lead people, one must also have charisma, energy, savvy, intelligence, and thick skin. Some leaders give orders, some work through opinion polls, and some plant thoughts into the minds of other people who can help them achieve their goals. Jack believes that a good deal is a good deal for everybody who is involved in the transaction. When the element of greed is eliminated from any venture, both sides win.

Some people emerge as giants by helping other people achieve their ambitions. Jack Anderson developed an intense desire to learn plastic surgery and to set a course which would not only help him achieve his personal goal, but would insure that any trained surgeon willing to "pay the price" could do so also.

It was for this reason that the American Academy of Facial Plastic and Reconstructive Surgery, Inc. was established. By his leadership, through his efforts, the Academy grew in numbers and credibility. Along the way, he has met tremendous resistance from competing specialty societies and surgeons who feel threatened by his ability, and has been singled out as someone who must be discredited.

At least one malpractice suit has been filed against him primarily because a general plastic surgeon in his community encouraged and assisted the plaintiff and his attorney. (More on that later.) Dr. Anderson was the lone individual singled out for attack by name in the article "Skim Milk Masquerades as Cream." Criticism from some is more honored than praise. In his leadership role, he has been attacked by his adversaries and praised by both his pupils and fellow facial plastic surgeons for what he has meant to his specialty. The results of national medical society elections suggest that he may be the most popular man within his specialty today, because he has fought off adversity and has helped others through hard times.

In the medical field, no one keeps a record of wins and losses, but I am convinced that he has meant to the specialty of *facial* plastic surgery what Coach Bryant meant to football. Dr. Jack Anderson is truly a giant among giants. His efforts will have a resounding effect upon plastic surgery for decades to come. My period of training with him certainly proved to be the spring-board to my career as a facial surgeon.

Berman

"Those who say it can't be done shouldn't interrupt those doing it."[3]

Our stay in the Beverly Hills area was fascinating. I was anxious to taste California. Susan had been there several years previously as Alabama's contestant in the Miss International Beauty Pageant (which has been replaced by the Miss Universe Pageant). She looked forward to returning there and reflecting upon some fond memories. We took advantage of the opportunity to see all the sights, and through Dr. Berman's facial plastic surgery practice, got to know many of the personalities of the "silver screen." Susan was a contestant on a television game show (Baffle) and studied skin care and make-up with Aida Grey in her plush Beverly Hills Beauty Salon. Wally and Dee made two Alabamians feel right at home in "Tinsel Town" (also the international center for cosmetic surgery).

Dr. Berman another former president of the American Academy of Facial Plastic and Reconstructive Surgery, is one of the founding members of the American Association of Cosmetic Surgeons. Through him I met Dr. Paul Ward, the chairman of the Department of Head and Neck Surgery at the UCLA Medical Center. At the conclusion of my training there, Dr. Ward offered me a position as the Director of the Section of Facial Plastic Surgery at UCLA. That opportunity was not only an honor, but was most appealing. Susan and I liked California. The people we had met there and the progressive nature of the medical community were intriguing.

Dr. Berman was a superb surgeon and had "weathered the storm" in the competitive Hollywood market, because he is good at what he does. As he had proven, cosmetic surgery was already firmly accepted as part of staying young and beautiful in the Los Angeles area. At that time I had some reservations about how it would be accepted in Birmingham. A few people from Birmingham were having cosmetic surgery done, but I discovered that many were going out-of-town for it (to New York, Miami or Arizona). I asked Dr. Ward for additional time to consider his offer. He agreed to keep it open.

---

[3]*Ibid*

The Continental Divide

After leaving California, we drove across the U.S.A. to Boston. The drive took five days. It gave us an opportunity to recognize the true magnificence of this great country. As we drove, we reflected, dreamed, and planned. Back-tracking the route taken by the early settlers who went west to establish a new way of life was an inspirational experience.

When we crossed the Continental Divide in Colorado, Susan and I realized that we were at a pivotal point in our lives, sitting on the edge of our past and the future. We both recognized the significance of the educational experience that was ours that year. I could not have become a facial surgeon without it.

Webster

"The happiest people are those who discover that what they should be doing and what they are doing are the same thing."[4]

The beauty and historical significance of Boston should give any patriotic American a warm feeling when he realizes how important that region was in shaping America's future. The time spent with Dr. Richard Webster certainly helped shape mine. It was more than I expected. Richard practiced a wide scope of facial and body plastic surgery. I think he is one of the most dynamic teachers I've found. His enthusiasm is infectious. Around him exists a kind of magnetism which draws a student closer and closer lest he miss some pearl of wisdom.

Dr. Webster is a pioneer who is secure enough in his own right to cross medical specialty picket lines to teach the skills of plastic surgery to head and neck (ENT) surgeons, dermatologists, ophthalmologists, oral surgeons, and others. He overcame attempts to discredit him by unfounded charges on his ethics and honesty as well as erroneous and malicious rumors about retirement, divorce and death.

---

[4]*Ibid*

Richard Webster has a dream,—to establish a specialty of "Cosmetic Surgery." It is happening. Today, he is the president and a founding member of the American Academy of Cosmetic Surgeons, Inc. Standing on the old north bridge outside Boston, one could almost hear "the shot fired around the world" and see the early American patriots charging across the open field to challenge the Redcoats head on. On the site where it all began, we realized more than ever that the brave men and women of the late 1700's were "giants" to whom each American owes so much. They had a dream, too. They put their lives on the line for our future. They chose to control their own destiny. Americans should never take for granted what they did as we enjoy the reality of their dream.

A Different Perspective

We left Boston pulling a U-Haul trailer in one of the most severe snowstorms that ever hit New England, barely escaping getting snowed in. Having traveled across this great land, and having lived in several geographic regions, we developed a different perspective of the United States of America. We came face to face with America's roots and our future. It was clear that people everywhere are just people. Some may look differently and speak with different dialects, but inside we are all simply human beings, passing through this world, each with his own set of dreams and problems. Often times we find in other people what we ourselves are searching.

There is a story of a man who, since he was a small boy, had a job operating the same piece of machinery at a small hometown factory. Hard times fell upon the factory and it closed. Knowing that he had to work, he set out to find another company that could utilize his services. He traveled from town to town looking for work and a new home. One day, he happened upon a group of elderly gentlemen sitting on a bench near the courthouse square of a small town. He approached the group and interrupted their conversation. "Say, old timer," he said, "What kind of people live in this town?" One of the gentlemen looked up at him and asked, "What kind of people lived in the town where you last lived?" He replied, "Kind, friendly and hardworking people." To his response, the old timer replied, "Then, if you look for them, that is the kind of people you will find here, my son."

There are good people, along with the bad, in every community.

As we go through everyday lives, we try to seek out those people who have similar goals, ideals, and ethics. Remember Young Boozer's mother's advice: "You can pick your friends. . ." Picking the right friends and role models is an important first step in being able to develop a life of fulfillment.

A Single Purpose

Isn't it a shame that we Americans allow ourselves to be divided up into sub-groups and that jealousy or envy causes us to expend energy against each other?

Bill Curry, the head football coach at Georgia Tech, recently told a group at the Birmingham Touchdown Club's father-son-daughter meeting, "If all people could spend some time on the football field in the huddle, we could all get along with each other better." In such a huddle people from all walks of life, black and white, rich and poor, smart and not-so-smart, come together with a single purpose and realize that by helping each other they can help themselves achieve personal goals.

During the broadcast of a national political convention, America saw the all-for-one, one-for-all tradition in jeopardy. It is bothersome to see forces attempting to fragment us—to destroy our "oneness."

Since our country's birth, Americans have pledged allegiance ". . .to one nation, under God, indivisible. . .," but, we saw an attempt at fragmentation into social, economic, racial, religious, and sexual subgroups in order to achieve self-serving political ambitions. It is contradictory to proclaim that repression of people's rights is intolerable, and then suggest that we should allow the injustice of communism to exist at our borders, inviting bondage. The communist's plan is clear. Nikita Khrushchev told us in the 1960's during a trip to the U.S., "We will bury you." Nothing since has changed. The Soviets meet with us to discuss peace only when it appears that we might be embarking upon some project which they want to thwart, like the "Star Wars" project. To date, their resolve has not changed, nor should ours.

Will American history books substitute Jesse Jackson's philosophy of "Peace is better than war and life is better than death" for the great American patriot Patrick Henry's "Give me liberty, or give me death," . . . or shall America's new motto become simply, "Give me?" We cannot afford to abandon the principles that have brought us to this point in history.

For how long . . . can so few . . . do so much . . . for so many? Americans have achieved prosperity through the work ethic, the strength of the family unit, and by placing their country's needs before individual desires. Such is the case with the players of any championship team.

We must stand committed to defeat any internal or external force which threatens our security . . . Can we afford to question the price tag of survival? Peace is best preserved through strength. John Kennedy said, "Let us never fear to negotiate, but let us never negotiate out of fear." Let us face the future with reason, not reaction; proven policies, not token politics; and confidence, not confusion. We must not allow ourselves to be deceived by the cunning or misled by the unknowing . . . to do either, will surely invite disaster. Too often, we get engulfed in our own set of problems and self-serving interests. Let us never forget the "mother lode."

The Collapse of Empires

Many historians have compared the Greek and Roman Empires to that of the United States of America. The concern is that the events which apparently led to their collapses can be seen all around us today. Some of the similarities between the rise to power and eventual decline of ours and those ancient civilizations were summarized in *The Rebirth of America*. In chronological order, they are:

1) Each civilization was built upon the foundation of a strong family unit.
2) Parents, not the state, accepted the responsibility of educating their children.
3) A strong work ethic produced a civilization of prosperity.
4) All three became nations of achievement. Each could boast of magnificent buildings, coliseums, and a vast network of roads and highways.
   What factors led to the beginning of the end?
1) As hired educators assumed the responsibilities of parents, the family unit disintegrated.

2) Family authority became delegated to big government, which attempted to "solve" the individual's problems.

3) Decline of morals was followed by the persecution of followers of The New Testament Church.

In the end, pagan Rome fell. The Greek civilization, which gave us Hippocrates and contributed much to our understanding of biology, philosophy, and anatomy, chose immorality and dependence upon government, rather than self, and collapsed shortly thereafter.

America still has a chance. It can choose the destiny of Rome and Greece or choose to return to the principles that have sustained us. It is a matter of choice.

The time spent in Boston gave us new insight into the values which were held so dearly by our country's founders. We cannot afford to forget from whence we came—America's genetics. Americans must not let a disruptive environment steer us in the wrong direction. History has divulged both the problem and the solution. Wise men and women need no more.

Three of the Best

When we arrived back in Alabama, I began to realize the benefits of that year's unique educational experience. We were bringing home increased wisdom and insight. Because of their willingness to share, I had been given an opportunity to experience through the medical practices of my teachers, in one year, what might have taken several years to learn from any of the more "traditional" routes.

By opening their offices and operating rooms to me, my facial plastic surgery teachers shared both their accomplishments and their problems. They passed to a young surgeon, eager to learn, what they themselves had learned through their experiences and from their teachers—the giants who had allowed them to see more clearly. I tried to load my wagon that year with bricks of pure gold. Hippocrates, the great physician, requested that, in dealing with each other, all future physicians "reckon (consider) him who taught me this art equally dear to me as my parents, to share my substance with him and . . . to teach . . . this art if they (other physicians) should wish to learn it . . . according to the law of medicine."

The word "doctor" means "teacher." Hippocrates would be proud

of Anderson, Berman and Webster (three giants), for they are truly
three of the best. They deserve to be honored by the Medical Hall of
Fame.

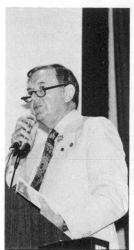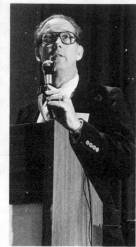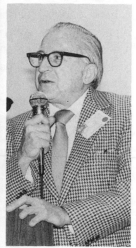

*Three "GIANTS": Jack R. Anderson, MD, Walter E. Berman, MD, and
Richard C. Webster, MD teaching at a plastic surgery seminar.*

CHAPTER 19

"CHOICE OF ALTERNATIVES"

Because I had been allowed to take my facial plastic fellowship during some of the time normally reserved only for residency training, Dr. Jim Hicks and I worked out an arrangement whereby I would stay on the teaching faculty at the University Hospital for a while and share with my fellow residents many of the things I had learned. That additional year also allowed me to obtain valuable surgical experience and to gain insight as a teacher.

Dr. John Kirklin

It was during this same time that another giant in the medical field would open some doors for me. Dr. John Kirklin, one of the world's premier heart surgeons, had recently left the Mayo Clinic to become the Chief of the Department of Surgery at the University Hospital. As a result of a challenge from some local plastic surgeons, it was necessary to ask that Dr. Kirklin grant me privileges to perform plastic surgery of the face at the University Hospital in Birmingham. He did. It was my first hospital staff appointment. His confidence was one of the key factors in my deciding to set up my practice in Birmingham.

Dr. Kirklin was a man who carried unparalleled respect in the

medical world because of his commitment to excellence. During the
time I studied under him, I had learned that he rarely took unwarranted risks. He and his staff could have performed a heart transplant
before Dr. Christian Barnard did in South Africa, but the chance of
the patient's body rejecting the transplanted heart was very high in
those days. Dr. Barnard's patient rejected the transplant and died.
It is my opinion that Dr. Kirklin considered the risk to the patient to
be too great—he demanded that the procedure carry a high proba-
bility of success before he would attempt it on his patient. Drawing
upon his wisdom, I have tried to carry this same philosophy into my
own practice.

It has been said that necessity is the mother of invention. Because
we are looking for something better, new procedures, cure-alls, gim-
micks, and devices frequently appear on the medical scene. Too
often, they fall by the wayside. Through expensive promotional campaigns, some corporations create public enthusiasm selling new devices and/or products, and some members of the medical profession,
trying to stay current, become trapped into using treatments that
later are found to be ineffective or potentially harmful.

Portrait of a Surgeon

In the early 1970's, the "distinguished lecturer" presentation was
awarded to Dr. Kirklin. He chose as his topic "Training Horses,
Quarterbacks, Pilots and Surgeons." Using experts in each of those
categories and carefully edited filmstrips, he demonstrated how it is
possible to teach a trainee to become an expert by the adoption of
constant standards, repetition, precision, and an unwavering commitment to excellence. Dr. Kirklin has graciously consented to my
sharing some of that presentation with the readers of this book. His
"surgeon" is a "cardiac surgeon." I believe his principles also apply
to any individual in training, be it medicine, business or athletics. He
said,

> "I've been struck by the similarities in the process of
> training the surgeon and that of training other types of liv-
> ing beings who may be doing very different things. These
> common denominators are interesting, and I confess that
> some of my own views of surgery, and of the teaching of

young people in the field, are borrowed from very different fields. . . Persons involved in surgery can function as a finely tuned team, just as do airline crews, horse and rider, and football teams.

You might ask "What is surgical knowledge?" The actual science and art of cutting and sewing, of finding tissue planes, of making repairs, and stopping hemorrhage, is just one of the things to be learned, but it must be mastered by the trainee. Some people ask, "What is there really to learn about doing surgery?" Before one begins to educate a surgeon, or a horse, or a quarterback or pilot, one must select the trainee. This selection process takes a considerable effort.

In surgery trainees, we look for intelligence and technical surgical aptitude, neither without the other being enough. We look for a *commitment to excellence* for without that the skills of the individual will never develop to have the brilliant focus required of the expert. We look for organizational ability, for the surgeon must have his rather complex and constantly changing knowledge and techniques always arranged so as to be instantly useful in potentially catastrophic emergencies. He must also be able to fit new knowledge and techniques in where they belong. He must also be able to form and maintain an effective surgical team. He must be able to interface effectively with colleagues in . . . other specialties. We look for good health and physical fitness, for surgery is physically demanding and one must be able when needed to work long hours without undue fatigue. We look for the staying power, inner strength and calm that will allow the individual to survive and thrive through a lifetime of surgery.

The young surgeon must have the self-confidence to proceed decisively on his own when necessary, and at the same time the humility to seek help and advice whenever possible. Some human qualities, integrity, self-appreciation without self-adulation, and true concern for people, eventually become a major determinant of a person's lifestyle. Although these may not impinge initially on his professional life, eventually they will. Now, no candidate possesses all of these ideal characteristics, but he must have the potential of developing all of them if he is to become and expert in this special kind of professional life.

If the candidate (for surgery training) happens also to have a sense of beauty and elegance, then he may be one of those rare pupils who some day will reach the pinnacles of surgery. For great surgery is elegant, and beautiful, with these coming in large part from perfection of technique and concept and a true striving for results and not effect. Such perfection of technique and concept not only in the operating room but also in pre- and postoperative evaluation and treatment, means that all is purposeful and unhurried, and no superfluous movement or word or piece of equipment or person mars the whole. The business man would say it is efficient, without waste of dollars or human resources. It is that, but also very much more. This kind of elegance results in a calm but efficient environment, facilitates learning and the development of new knowledge, and assures superior surgical care for the patient, which of course is the endpoint of the whole affair."

Dr. Kirklin's presentation and his philosophy served as a cornerstone in helping me define my own personal surgical goals, in the establishment of the McCollough Facial Surgry Clinic, P.A., and in the fellowship training program which we offer to young facial surgeons in cooperation with The American Academy of Facial Plastic and Reconstructive Surgery, Inc. Quality is the key to longevity—a thing that seems to have lost significance in America's marketplace.

> *"Quality is never an accident; it is always the result of high intention, sincere effort, intelligent direction and skillful execution; it represents the wise choice of many alternatives."*[1]

The "choice of alternatives" is what this book is all about.

---

[1] Willa A. Foster, *Motivational Quotes* p. 74.

"Big Ruby Gets Facelift"

One of my early surgical cases created quite a fracas. It led to the decision about my staff appointment and surgical privileges having to be made earlier than anticipated. A choice of alternatives had to be made by Dr. Kirklin and by me.

Upon returning to Alabama from my facial plastic fellowship training, Dr. Hicks introduced me to Governor George Wallace's former mother-in-law, Mrs. Ruby Folsom (Big Ruby). She wanted to have a facelift. Dr. Hicks had her wait for me to return so that I could perform her surgery. The surgery was scheduled and performed at the University Hospital. She was happy with the results and told almost everyone with whom she came in contact about her surgery and her surgeon. Ruby is not bashful. She did for facial plastic surgery in Alabama what Phyllis Diller did throughout America.

I was still a resident at the University Hospital when I did her surgery. She told a newspaper reporter during an interview of her daughter, Cornelia Wallace (George's former wife), about her surgery. The reporter divulged the entire story about her surgery in the article she was writing about Cornelia. Ruby truly thought she was doing me a favor. Maybe in the long run she did, because this incident brought important issues to the surface quickly.

A few days later, The *Birmingham News* carried an article entitled, "Big Ruby Gets Facelift." That article upset a number of the *general* plastic surgeons in Birmingham. Because of the incident, Dr. Kirklin, as Chief of Surgery, had to make some decisions. There were two major problems. First, at the time I performed the surgery I was still classified as a resident and therefore, had not *officially* completed my full course of training. Secondly, my prescribed course of training in FACIAL PLASTIC SURGERY differed from that of the *general* plastic surgeons. That fact was a BIG deal, to them.

Dr. Kirklin's decision would become a key factor in determining where I was ultimately going to live and practice. Would Alabama be willing to recognize the evolutionary change which had occurred in the delivery of plastic surgery by specialists in head and neck (ENT) surgery? It had already occurred in other states.

I still had the option to return to UCLA as the director of the section of Facial Plastic Surgery—a tempting offer. After months of vacillating between Birmingham and Beverly Hills, the choice became clear. I asked myself, "What does anyone want out of life?" I concluded that if one has a place to practice his profession, a good place to rear his family, and a group of devoted friends, he has what he needs. I concluded that all those things were here in Alabama. It seemed foolish to pull up my roots and move across the country looking for the very things I already had. Like most dilemmas, complex problems usually have simple solutions.

The decision was made. I would plow new ground at home and roll with the tide of changes occurring within my field of medicine.

Putting on a New Face

The changing face of our specialty was outlined by Dr. Jack Anderson during a presentation to the Southern Medical Association. The title of the presentation was "An Old Medical Specialty Puts On a New Face . . . and Head . . . and Neck." In the article, he concluded that,

> "A quiet evolution had occurred in one of medicine's most venerable specialties, the second to organize an American board for certification purposes.

> "Otolaryngology has acquired an identity that clearly reflects its transformation from an organ specialty (ear, nose and throat) into a modern regional specialty encompassing otolaryngology AND head and neck medicine and surgery."

> "Involvement of the otolaryngologist in plastic and maxillofacial surgery has been of long standing. In 1888, Rowe, an otolaryngologist of Rochester, New York, reported the first nasal plastic procedure (rhinoplasty) without using external incisions. An otolaryngologist was among the founding members of the American Board of Plastic Surgery in 1939, 14 years after formation of the American Board of Otolaryngology. The man considered to be the father of plastic surgery in all circles, Sir Harold Gilles, was an otolaryngologist—an ENT specialist."

> "Since the time of Rowe, otolaryngologists have used plastic procedures whenever necessary in their work.

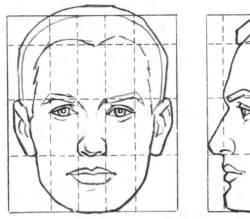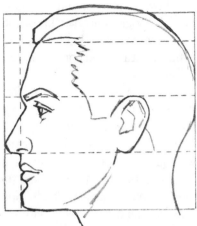

Leonardo da Vinci's "ideal" facial proportions are demonstrated by these diagrams.

Such methods have been applied in their ear surgery, to shift tissues, to correct deformities caused by cancers they have removed, to repair congenital deformities (birth defects), and to provide functional and cosmetic improvement in the face, nose, head and neck."

"The young surgeon training in otolaryngology gains a special competence in head and neck plastic and reconstructive surgery, because he is more familiar with the anatomy, physiology, and pathology of that region than someone who is not trained in the area or who works there only occasionally."

A New, More Fitting Identity

Since specialization was first recognized in medicine, there has been a trend toward regionalization, or confining one's work to a specific anatomic region of the body.

Otolaryngologists have traditionally been designated as the ear, nose, and throat (or ENT) specialty. The scope of other medical specialists are much better understood by the public, and by the rest of the medical profession. Ob-gyn specialists, for example, are not called ovary, uterus, and vagina men, nor is the specialty known as OUV. Urologists are not known as kidney, ureter, and bladder men, nor is the specialty known as KUB. Neurosurgeons are not known as nerve, brain, and cord men, nor is their specialty known as NBC.

Certainly the letters "ENT" or the words, "ear, nose and throat" do not encompass the other major surgical procedures performed by these specialists in the head and neck including: face lifting (rhytidectomy), eyelid plastic surgery (blepharoplasty), nasal plastic surgery (rhinoplasty), hair transplantation, chemical peeling, dermabrasion, facial implants, scar revision, repair of facial injuries or reconstruction of cancer and tumor defects of the forehead, scalp, cheeks, major salivary glands, lips and oral cavity, and the correction of numerous birth defects within the face, head and neck.

Superspecialization

The specialty (Otolaryngology—Head and Neck Surgery) lends itself to superspecialization such as facial plastic surgery. It was the recognition of this evolutionary process that made me elect to pursue this course of training as the foundation for my career as a facial surgeon. It appeared my destiny. It certainly was my choice.

Dr. Kirklin had to make a decision, one that might "pinch some toes." Was Alabama ready to accept this evolutionary process? If not, I still had a couple of "aces in the hole." The offer from UCLA to head up a section of facial plastic surgery in Los Angeles was there, or I could return to New Orleans to practice with Dr. Anderson, one of my mentors. Both of those were win-win situations.

A Turning Point

After weeks of deliberation—an examination of the facts—Dr. Kirklin ruled in my favor. He made it clear to me, and others, that it was because of my interest and special training in the field of facial plastic surgery that the opportunity to do this work at the University Hospital was available to me. That decision became a turning point in Birmingham medical politics because, prior to that time, only *general* plastic surgeons were permitted to do many of the cosmetic plastic surgical procedures in most hospitals in the city. I believe that his decision opened doors for many *specialty* plastic surgeons who had received the appropriate training to perform the same procedures.

Callahan Had a Vision

In order to furthur develop my practice in facial plastic surgery, I also needed to be on the staff of a smaller, private hospital, so I contacted the founder of the Eye Foundation Hospital, Dr. Alston Callahan, an eye plastic surgeon. I had worked there as a medical student (one of my many moonlighting jobs) doing pre-operative screening for patients who were undergoing eye surgery. Dr. Callahan and I had previously talked about my doing a residency in ophthalmology (eye specialist) before I decided to go into facial surgery.

The Eye Foundation Hospital was established against great resistance and professional jealousy. Dr. Callahan had overcome adversity and assaults on both his personal and professional integrity. He outworked his critics and ascended to international prominence as the man who "wrote the book" on ophthalmic plastic surgery.

When I needed his help, Dr. Callahan agreed to support my application to the staff.

Today the Eye Foundation Hospital stands in the heart of the UAB Medical Center as a tribute to this man who had a vision.

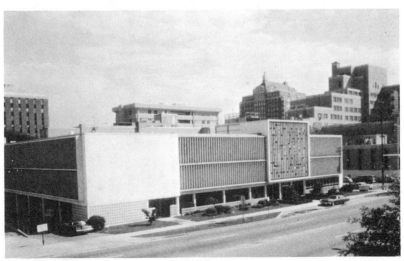

The Eye Foundaton Hospital (Callahan's vision) in the heart of the UAB Medical Center.

PART IV

"WHAT MEN DARE DO"

CHAPTER 20

THE PLASTIC SURGERY "COLD WAR"

"Difficulty is an instructor. He that wrestles with us strengthens our nerves and sharpens our skills. Our antagonist is our helper. . ."[1]

I hoped I could prevent the national interspecialty conflict from becoming a problem in Alabama. Naively, I felt if I could meet with two of the *general* plastic surgeons who were my teachers during medical school, internship, or surgical residency, that the three of us could work to prevent a conflict from developing on the local level.

Upon returning to Alabama from my fellowship, I called them and asked for a meeting. When the meeting took place they scoffed at my facial plastic surgical training and informed me, in no uncertain terms, that they had no interest in working with me. Measures could be taken to make it difficult for me to establish my practice in the Birmingham community. One of them said he was a member of an important committee at the Baptist Medical Center—Montclair, a hospital where I had served my internship, and would try to see that I was prevented from performing facial plastic surgery there. (Brook-

---

[1]Burk, *Treasury of Familiar Quotations* p. 78.

wood Hospital had not been built.) The other degraded some of my teachers, then gave me an emotional lecture on being a *general* plastic surgeon, a career route I had seriously considered and discarded after consulting with him when he was on the staff at the University Hospital. He had discouraged me from going into general plastic surgery—an interesting turnabout. In 1968, he recommended I look into kidney transplantation instead—no competition to a general plastic surgeon. My interest was in becoming a facial surgeon not a body plastic surgeon, and certainly not a kidney transplant surgeon.

We had decided to go in different directions. I had made my choice. I became board-certified to do *facial* plastic surgery by the American Board of Otolaryngology, representing the specialty of Head and Neck Surgery. I had also successfully completed an approved fellowship by the American Academy of Facial Plastic and Reconstructive Surgery, Inc. I had not come asking for these two general plastic surgeon's approval or blessings. I thought I was coming as a former student, friend, and peacemaker. At least I learned where I stood with them. On that day in 1974, they made it clear that at least where they were concerned, friendship ended where business began. How ridiculous, I thought, for surgeons to admit they would campaign against a fellow surgeon, much less a former student (remember Hippocrates). That was their choice. I had already made mine. They went to work and so did I. Down through the years the facts about my training and board-certification have been twisted by ill-wishers to make it look as though I have misrepresented my credentials. I did not anticipate seeing professionals use tactics non-becoming a professional.

Henry Yielding wrote, "The slander of some people is as great a recommendation as the praise of others."[2] More on that theme later.

I hadn't come to these two plastic surgeons looking for a battle. I also wasn't looking to get hit by mud-slinging. I simply wanted to practice my skills in an atmosphere of mutual respect and cooperation. Quickly, I realized that I was starting my drive in the shadows of my own goal posts. If it was going to be a "gut-check", I had survived them before; therefore, the challenge did not weaken my commitment. Maybe the adversity I met drove me into trying to be a better surgeon.

---

[2]*Seeds To Sow* p. 56.

Plato advised, "When men speak ill of thee, live so nobody may believe them." Truth prevails.

"Restraint of Trade"

Now, I'm going to take you into the inner sanctum of the medical profession—an examination of the *national* dispute between the practitioners of plastic surgery. The report will shock many of you. It is, however, part of the story that needs to be told.

Several years after that meeting, I realized that the conflict between the *general* plastic surgeons and *specialty* plastic surgeons was of a long-standing, well-conceived nature, seemingly initiated by some *general* plastic surgeons.

One document from the files of the American Society of Plastic and Reconstructive Surgeons called it a "cold war." Because of suspected anti-competitive activities, the Federal Trade Commission initiated an investigation of the *general* plastic surgeons' national organization (The American Society of Plastic and Reconstructive Surgeons). The plastic surgeons' counsel apparently felt that enough evidence had been uncovered during the investigation that a consent agreement was signed and offered to the Federal Trade Commission by the executive director and legal counsel of ASPRS. As I understand it, this indicates that the general plastic surgeons were afraid of losing.

In the consent agreement, the general plastic surgeons' national organization (ASPRS) offered to *"cease and desist* from engaging in any activity . . . which has the purpose or effect of depriving, foreclosing, limiting or restricting any non-ASPRS physician's access to:

(1) participation in the treatment or surgery of patients hospitalized for plastic and reconstructive surgery;
(2) hospital privileges to perform plastic and reconstructive surgery;
(3) use of the word "plastic" or "plastic surgeon" to describe a field of medical practice;
(4) telephone or other directory listings;
(5) instruction by members of ASPRS or physicians certified by ABMS;
(6) educational programs; and

(7) publication of advertisements or announcements in any publications other than ASPRS publications."

The fact that a consent agreement existed has not been generally disclosed.

From the Federal Trade Commission and through the Freedom of Information Act, another document was uncovered from the files of the American Society of Plastic and Reconstructive Surgeons which outlined a plan for dealing with other medical specialties that also performed plastic surgery. In it, the general plastic surgeons' executive vice-president anticipated that their anti-competitive activities established as far back as 1975 might ultimately lead to a "restraint of trade" action against them.

The following excerpts represent the tenor of the document

". . . we (the general plastic surgeons) have the power, ability and cohesiveness of our members to *stall* and *frustrate* the majority of their (facial plastic surgeons) efforts. . ." (emphasis added)

". . . In particular, it could reach a point of legal vulnerability that would lead to *restraint of trade* action. . ." (emphasis added)

". . . We (general plastic surgeons) must go back to the original concepts that allowed this group (facial surgeons) to grow and appreciate our ability to have *frustrated their efforts* as long as we have. . ." (emphasis added)

". . . We must plan a course of action that will allow us to stall as long as we can, *neutralize their* (facial surgeons) *leadership*. . ." (Later we shall review some tactics they may have used to "*neutralize*" the leadership of the facial plastic surgeons) (emphasis added)

". . . We (the general plastic surgeons) need to evaluate all options before moving into conflict resolution on a purely agressive posture by seeking to *destroy* or *further suppress* this outgroup (facial surgeons). . ." (emphisis added)

The use of words like "*power*," "*stall*," "*frustrate*," "*neutralize*," "*to destroy or furthur suppress*" have no place in American medicine.

One of the documents uncovered by The Federal Trade Commission during its investigation of the general plastic surgeons outlined a plan consisting of establishing a "cold war" strategy based upon the principles of "Fabian Socialism." The document also described a plan to establish teams "to handle guerrilla warfare break-outs" and to establish a public relations program designed to offset any public recognition of *facial* plastic surgeons. The *general* plastic surgeons would attempt to thwart many of the inroads being made by other specialties by waging their "own form of cold war." (In Chapter 22, we shall review how one form of cold war is conducted). The fact that such a "plan" existed in which one medical specialty would attempt to discredit another has been an embarrassment to the entire medical profession.

In Mark Twain's autobiography he concluded that,

> "of all creatures that were made, he (man) is the most detestable. Of the entire brood, he is the one—the solitary one—that possesses malice. . . He is the only creature that inflicts pain for sport, knowing it to *be* pain. . . Also in all the list, he is the only creature with a nasty mind."

Because a group of *general* plastic surgeons in Georgia may have stepped over the boundaries of the law, a $10 million libel suit has been filed against The Georgia Society of Plastic and Reconstructive Surgeons and two of its leaders (Drs. Rusca and Huger) who listed themselves as authors of a defamatory article which was published in the journal of the state medical society representing physicians from all specialties throughout the state of Georgia. In that article, the *general* plastic surgeons claimed that *they* were "cream" and that other surgeons performing plastic surgery and who did not belong to the general plastic surgeons' organizations were "skim milk" and lacked credentials. The *general* plastic team may have violated the rules. The courts will determine if they did, and if they will be penalized for "unsportsmanlike conduct."

Because it was felt that the "skim milk article" was an example of libel against the parties specifically named in the article, the American Academy of Facial Plastic and Reconstructive Surgeons, the American Association of Cosmetic Surgeons and Dr. Jack R. Anderson, all three injured parties, filed suit against the *general* plastic surgeons who were credited for the article.

Many examples exist around the country where *general* plastic surgeons attempted to prevent facial or *specialty* plastic surgeons who are also "board-certified" from being admitted to hospital staffs and kept off emergency room call lists. I think that's restraint of trade. It certainly strains the ethics of medicine and violates the Hippocratic Oath. I don't believe you help people rise up by tearing the achievers down.

Katz vs Anderson

Why was Dr. Anderson singled out in the "skim milk" article? In 1973, a lawsuit for "malpractice" was tried in the U.S. District Court of New Orleans against Dr. Jack R. Anderson.

At the trial, a plastic surgeon was brought in from out of state to testify against Dr. Anderson. Of note, are the following facts:

1.) The leading local plastic surgical witness against Dr. Anderson was Dr. Robert Ryan, chairman of the Public Relations Committee of the American Society of Plastic and Reconstructive Surgeons and chairman of Plastic Surgery at Tulane University. He competed with Dr. Anderson for patients.

2.) The same "local plastic surgeon," (Ryan) had tried to actively stop an educational seminar which was given by facial plastic surgeons in 1968 in New Orleans.

3.) Two months after the patient saw Ryan, the patient instituted the suit.

4.) Ryan had personally lined up the out-of-state plastic surgical witness (who was an attorney as well as a general plastic surgeon) to come testify against Dr. Anderson.

5.) After seeing the patient, Ryan had written a letter to Dr. Anderson stating that he felt the plaintiff (Katz) did not have a basis for a medical malpractice suit.

6.) Ryan sat in the courtroom throughout most of the trial and appeared to advise the plaintiff's attorney. He also testified against Dr. Anderson.

7). The patient has since given a sworn statement that Dr. Ryan directed the litigation, that the patient was told he would not have to pay anything for the lawsuit, and that the general plastic surgeons had been looking for a plaintiff. In retrospect, the patient stated, he believed the general plastic surgeons would like very much to remove Dr. Anderson's group (facial plastic surgeons) from that type of practice.

If Dr. Anderson, the leading proponent of *facial* plastic surgery, could be nailed for using the words "plastic surgery," then the *general* plastic surgeons would have gone a long way to discourage and discredit other regional specialists.

The court saw through the smokescreen. Dr. Anderson won the case.

How do I know these things? I was *there* doing my fellowship at the time. The eyes of an aspiring young surgeon were opened to an interspecialty conflict extending beyond New Orleans. That's why I asked for a meeting with two general plastic surgeons I knew when I came back to Birmingham after completing my fellowship. I had seen what had happened in New Orleans and in other cities. Naively, I had hoped I could prevent it in Birmingham. I was wrong.

It is likely that other malpractice suits have been initiated against competing *specialty* plastic surgeons by *general* plastic surgeons. I was asked to review a case in Birmingham which I believe was filed based upon statements made by a general plastic surgeon against treatment rendered by a local ENT surgeon.

In the face of a malpractice insurance crisis, it is despicable to think that one physician would intentionally initiate a malpractice suit against another as part of an interspecialty "cold war," try to make life difficult for a competing surgeon, or to try to shift blame to a fellow physician.

It is a different matter if the physician practices in a way which might endanger the health, safety and welfare of his patients. *Most* physicians are trying to do something to help solve the malpractice crisis.

In today's society, one would think that anti-competitive activities, slander and libel, would be recognized as such serious offenses that anyone would be reluctant to risk the consequences.

Shakespeare wrote, "O, what men dare do! What men may do! What men daily do, knowing not what they do." I have been shocked at what some "dare do." Many function at the brink dividing good and evil, right from wrong, legal and illegal.

Alabama's Law

The offenders who "dare do," may know "not what they do." In Alabama, the law clearly states. . .

> "one who repeats or otherwise republishes defamatory matter is subject to liability as if he had originally published it." The law treats the speaker of a slanderous remark as liable, even if he "accompanies the slander with a statement that it is a rumor only, or designates the name of the author as the original publisher."

This rule is applicable although the listener may have already heard similar statements from other sources.

Some of the problems I have faced in Birmingham looked like part of a coordinated national campaign against all facial and *specialty* plastic surgeons who are "board-certified" either by The American Boards of Otolaryngology (Head and Neck Specialists), Opthalmology (Eye Specialists) and Dermatology (Skin Specialists). My local problems may be simply sniper attacks or minor acts of a kind of terrorism being directed, or at least encouraged, from a higher level.

Having been trained on the athletic battlefields, the resistance seemed to make my commitment to succeed stronger. I thought back to the fourth down play on the goal line in the Orange Bowl and Coach Bryant's comments following the play. Trying to leave no room for doubt and believing that the public, not a competitor with an ax to grind, is the ultimate judge of surgical competence, I set out to establish my practice.

Medical Chauvinism

In 1986, for selfishly-motivated surgeons to proclaim that *only they* possess the necessary skills to do certain facial procedures seems narrow-minded. Chauvinism is defined by *The American Heritage Dictionary* as the "prejudiced belief in the superiority of one's own

group." For anyone to be so fanatically impressed with his own educational degree is reminiscent of Benjamin Franklin's statement,
"Tim was so learned that he could name a horse in nine languages;
. . . (but) . . . he bought a cow to ride on."

The American Medical Association, the American College of Surgeons and the American Hospital Association all recognize and have
recommended that surgeons from several specialties can, and
should, perform the same surgical procedures. Because the *general*
plastic surgeons apparently wish to thwart competition through public relations campaigns and private conversations, they have tried to
sell the public on the idea that *only* those surgeons who are members
of *their* organizations are qualified to perform plastic surgery. In their
advertisements, the *general* plastic surgeons advise the public not to
consult anyone except one of their members. Hundreds of thousands
of dollars are spent annually on such advertising campaigns.

Until yet, no one has measured the damage done by cocktail party
and locker room loose talk designed to defame and slander competing
surgeons. In the near future, a jury may reach for the scales of justice to measure the amount of damage inflicted by malicious tongues
and reckless pens.

The Facts

In the booklet, "Delineation of Hospital Privileges for the Practice
of Head and Neck Plastic Surgery" (AAFPRS), the facts are clearly
summarized:

> "In the area of head and neck surgery, the practice of head
> and neck **plastic** surgery is sometimes misunderstood.
> This is due largely to the fact that decision makers tend to
> think of plastic surgery as a *specialty* rather than a *method*
> of surgery."

This is as ridiculous as claiming that only the quarterback should
be able to run with the football. The "ball carrier" is not a designated
position on the team—it is any player who advances the ball. If he can
score touchdowns, who cares what number he wears on his jersey.

William "Refrigerator" Perry of the Chicago Bears may have
started a whole new trend in short yardage situations in football. He

wears number 72, an unlikely number to score touchdowns, but he gets the job done. A few foolish souls have tried to convince him that he shouldn't carry the ball. His record speaks. He can, should and does score touchdowns.

When the doctor in the emergency room carefully sutures a cut on the face with fine delicate sutures, he is performing "plastic" surgery. When the orthopedic surgeon reconstructs a hand which has been mangled in an industrial accident, he is performing "plastic" surgery. When the neurosurgeon repairs a defect in the skull following a motorcycle accident, he is performing "plastic" surgery and when the oral surgeon repositions a protruding jaw, he is performing "plastic" surgery. A "plastic surgeon" then could be defined as "a surgeon who performs plastic surgery."

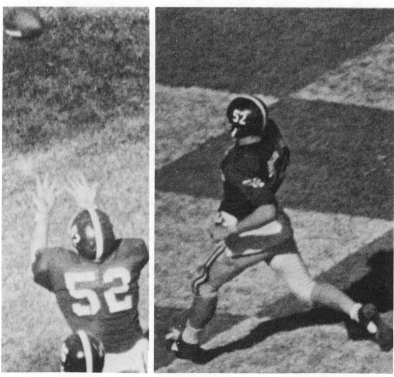

An offensive center (Gaylon McCollough) fields a blocked punt and carries the ball into the Tennessee end zone (Alabama vs Tennessee, 1964) for a touchdown. Number 52, an unlikely number to score touchdowns.

"Plastic surgery may be performed in all areas of the body
by a *general* plastic surgeon, or in areas of specialty practice by a *specialty* plastic surgeon.[3]

The practice of regional plastic surgery within the various specialties has advanced over the years with the trend toward medical
specialism. Overlapping clinical interests of physicians are here to
stay, but some "traditional" plastic surgeons refuse to accept the
inevitable.

Victor Hugo once said "there is one thing stronger than all the
armies in the world, and that is an idea whose time has come."

Superspecialization and anatomic regionalization of the practice of
medicine and surgery is an "idea whose time has come." Today, we
have hand surgeons, heart surgeons, eye surgeons, ear surgeons,
facial surgeons, and head and neck surgeons. The generalists in
medicine have a right to feel threatened. They could choose, however, to select a specific area of their field and concentrate their efforts on improving their knowledge and skills in order to become
better surgeons (and stop bellyaching).

The true test of competence for any specialists lies in the quality
of work performed over a period of time, whether the person doing
the work be black or white, tall or short, man or woman. Can the individual get the job done? That is the question. No individual, no organization, no single certifying board can honestly proclaim or
legislate a monopoly on competence and knowledge. To do so is chauvinism in its purest form. In my daily practice, I see the results of
surgery performed by plastic and reconstructive surgeons from
many areas of the country. Some patients come to have correction of
unsuccessful surgery performed by the very surgeons who protest
most loudly. Should I wish to stoop so low, I could plant the seed for
a malpractice suit against at least one of my competitors each week.
A surgeon who claims that he has *no* complications is either not performing any surgery, is not following his patients closely enough after
surgery, operates by a different set of standards, or is lying.

About Proclamation

Once, a delegation of "advisors" visited President Lincoln and
urged that he declare emancipation before he was ready. He knew

---

[3]AAFPRS, *Delineation of Hospital Privileges.*

the timing was all wrong and argued that he could not enforce it even if he proclaimed it. To the group Lincoln asked, "How many legs will a sheep have if you call the tail a leg?" "Five," they answered. "You are mistaken," said Lincoln, "for calling a tail a leg don't make it so." Likewise, claiming to be the only authority on a subject "don't make it so" either.

The American Medical Association which speaks for the physician community has concluded that physicians representing several specialties can and should be permitted to perform the same procedures.

The AMA has tried to help resolve the interspecialty conflict by developing a joint statement arrived at from the input of both the *general* and the head and neck (plastic) surgeons. Hopefully, one day soon, a truce will be signed. The conflict between medical specialties must come to an end, one way or the other. The scales of justice and reason must be brought back into balance.

Live and Let Live

Americans function in a tremendously educated society. The average high school senior knows more about the physical laws of the universe, DNA, genetics, and the principles of "high tech" than the greatest scientist of a century ago. With all this knowledge about our universe, people have not yet learned how to get along with each other. There are too many barriers which pit human beings against each other.

Today, man exists in both organizational and individual frameworks. Certain standards of behavior which are acceptable in one, are taboo in the other. The human race is developing a "split personality"—a type of social schizophrenia.

In the organizational framework, a group of individuals act together driven by a common cause. Organizations often provide security, and allow the individual to function in a way which he could not achieve independently. On the other hand, he often participates in organizational misbehavior that he would never consider, individually. He finds strength in numbers. The "little man" Napoleon complex is bolstered by being a part of an army of colleagues with similar interests. When the individual leaves the organizational framework, he reverts to more primitive behavior and lives by a different, more liberal set of rules.

Organizational leaders know how to manipulate individual behavior. If man would reverse this thought process and begin to make organizations, governments, political parties and religions revert to individual standards, conflicts could be reduced to simple, resolvable issues.

American medicine has too many problems with which to contend to allow turf battles to divide its ranks. Either cooler heads must prevail, or the referees (the courts) shall decide the issue, in which case, both sides will more than likely emerge as losers. Only the lawyers will win.

When both sides of the plastic surgery conflict realize that each is firmly entrenched, will not go away or back down, has the necessary manpower and resources, and the commitment to survive, as is the case with nuclear war, peace is the ONLY alternative.

Following a long and bloody battle, a General approached his Ruler and proclaimed—"I have the honor, your Imperial Highness, to announce a great victory." "Very well," the Ruler said, "Go and congratulate your troops." The General replied, "There are none left."[4]

Tolerance is a better solution than annihilation. If the current practice of disparagement, slander and libel persists, physicians can eventually mortally wound each other in the courtrooms. Only the lawyers will win. Live and let live—the violators must be brought back in line, otherwise, the risks are too great for either side.

Dealing with Conflict

One might wonder why I have spent so much time reviewing the conflict between two medical societies that perform plastic surgery.

Firstly, I have tried to set the record straight. I believe when the public knows the facts about the issues and the players, both sides may lay the gauntlet aside. Then surgeons can get on with improving their skills and caring for patients.

Secondly, it is a major problem that I have had to deal with both personally and professionally. In doing so, I have been forced to reach deep into my soul and draw upon the strength and wisdom of those whose opinions I respect: to apply the principles of dealing with conflict that fill the book shelves of the world. I have been challenged to

---

[4]*Anecdotes* p. 424.

carry the lessons learned upon the field of athletics into the game of life.

Thirdly, similar conflicts exist throughout the business and professional world. There are no new problems. One only needs to change the names, dates, and places and the story might be the same. I hope each person who reads this book will examine the conflicts herein described. In the final analysis, you should gain some insight into your own problems by realizing that yours are similar to those encountered by others, both mortals and giants.

The "Cold War" Must End

In the fall of 1986, I shall be installed as the President of the American Academy of Facial Plastic and Reconstructive Surgery, Inc., the organization which represents almost 3,000 *specialty* plastic surgeons throughout most of the free world. During that year, I would like to see the beginning of the end of the interspecialty conflict. I wonder if, like the Arab-Israeli, and USA-USSR conflicts, there is a peaceful solution. The two specialties must begin to seek peace and harmony. "Cold War" has no place in American medicine. It must not be passed to the next generation of surgeons who do not yet know about the conflict which has plagued us and our predecessors. Once informed, I do not believe that you, the public, will allow it to continue. You can tell your doctor to stop talking about a colleague and talk to you about the problem for which you have consulted him. That's what you are paying him for. Had you been looking for gossip, you could have chosen less expensive places. You also wouldn't have had to wait for two hours to get to the source.

Little did I know that so much of a physician's energies could become wrapped up in dealing with non-medical problems. Maybe that's the way it has always been. Hopefully, that's not the way it will always be. I'd like to see those energies used to make life better rather than creating problems for each other. Then there would be no need for "referees."

During my term as president of the American Academy of Facial Plastic and Reconstructive Surgery, I hope that I shall be able to draw upon the wisdom of great minds and the sanity of prudent leaders of the two involved medical specialties so that together we can merge our energies, knowledge, and experience to establish a stronger foundation for the surgeons of tomorrow.

Not every plastic surgeon has been involved in or supported the "cold war." I believe that Dr. Luis Vasconez, chairman of plastic surgery at UAB, and I have developed a professional and educational relationship that can lead to cooperation and mutual respect—there are others, too. Like we once did, our students are looking for role models. The ultimate winner in such a combined effort will be our patients. If physicians do these things, the losers will be our lawyers. The "Cold War" must end! The solution to war is no more war. Then, both the general plastic surgeons and the specialty plastic surgeons are victors. Professional cooperation can only lead to improving the knowledge and skills of all surgeons performing plastic surgery. The future of plastic surgery in America is a destiny of choice.

As a consumer, I challenge the medical profession to stop bellyaching and choose a course of excellence. Make good things happen. Cast troublemakers aside and provide the quality of care we, the public, deserve in a spirit of cooperation.

CHAPTER 21

FACING ADVERSITY

"To escape criticism—do nothing, say nothing, be nothing"[1]

I guess the corollary to that is if one plans to do nothing and be nothing he should live a quiet non-controversial life. If becoming the first facial surgeon in Alabama to establish an independent outpatient clinic was to be my goal, then I should have been prepared for criticism. It came from all directions and from several camps. Each day I read Rudyard Kipling's "If" and tried to keep things in perspective. I became immersed in my work. I could control what I did; I could not control what adversaries were saying.

In writing this book, I am violating the "say nothing" part of the above quotation. I have said something about my heroes, my adversaries, my country, my profession, my family, my community, myself, and my dream for a destiny that I believe is obtainable. Some will take offense to what I have written. If, however, some find this book beneficial, my efforts have been worthwhile.

As we have recognized, the game of life is tough, fraught with peaks and valleys. One spends a third of his life preparing for his career, a third working in his chosen profession and about a third in retirement reflecting upon what he did or did not do. Completion of

---

[1] Elbert Hubbard, *Peter's Quotations* p. 144.

one's formal educational program does not mean that he has scored in life's game. He has simply made a first down and is provided an opportunity to make another first down, and another, until he scores. If he chooses to do so, he can continue running up the score in the game of life until the final buzzer sounds. When it's all over, hopefully, he can be inducted into the Hall of Fame that really counts.

Until that time, nothing can be taken for granted.

Just when the game seems to be under control, drastic events happen. In 1972, Auburn won a football game from Alabama (17-16) on two blocked punts at the end of a game Auburn hadn't even been in. In life, too, strange things can happen when people try to block our efforts to advance. The lessons learned from athletics help prepare us for what lies ahead.

Dare to be Different

Once the decision had been made as to where I would establish my practice, the next step would be to develop a long range plan and to assemble my team. I knew that it would take the same kind of effort to build a successful facial surgery practice that I had seen succeed in athletics. From the outset, my destination was different from that which had already been established. That fact was not a problem. Someone once said, "Do not follow where the path may lead. Go instead where there is no path and leave a trail."[2]

I had learned that first one must have a well-defined image of what he hopes to achieve. Establishing a long-range goal was the second step. Next, it would be necessary to surround myself with a staff of competent, dedicated people. Then, I would try to improve my technical skills each day in order to become a little better with each surgical experience. The plan would be to incorporate the lessons learned in athletics—work harder than my competitors. The philosophy at my clinic would be to treat people as I would like to be treated if doctor-patient roles were reversed. My team would be committed to the pursuit of excellence as outlined by Dr. Kirklin in his "Distinguished Lecturer" presentation.

I had seen this approach work in winning traditions at Enterprise and at the University of Alabama and felt sure that it could apply to

---

[2]Anonymous, *Motivational Quotes* p. 19.

the business and professional world as well. I knew it would be necessary to make decisions and live with the consequences. Some actions would, by necessity, be unpopular. Because my plan was to establish something which threatened "the establishment," I was certain to "pinch some toes," but I accepted the challenge. This was *my* dream. No other person could fight this battle for me, nor did I want one to. Like Lindbergh's flight across the Atlantic, the trip would be fraught with risks, but the destination was clear. I was at the controls. David Seabury once said,

> *"Don't worry about the whole world: if you do, it will overwhelm you . . . Please yourself. Do something for you, and the rest will fall in line."*[3]

On June 4, 1986, the Alabama Public Broadcasting System aired a special on the life of a little known 19th century American artist, Thomas Akins. One hundred years later his work has emerged as the standard by which painters compare their skills. His best painting, "The Gross Clinic," is a true-to-life depiction of an operation being performed in a teaching ampitheater by the world famous surgeon, Dr. Samuel Gross. Akin's work was ridiculed by his 19th century critics. He was ostrasized by his countemporaries and driven into seclusion by untrue rumors of immorality.

"The Gross Clinic" initially sold for only $200. Today, it is worth millions. In his entire life Akins sold only twenty paintings. He was unable to give some of his works away.

Akins knew he was good at what he did. That fact drove him to continue doing what he did best. He was ahead of his time, a threat to the establishment. Today, the genius of Thomas Akins is acclaimed by an art world which disparaged him during his lifetime.

Change is most often met with resistance. Throughout history, innovators have been chastised by much of the establishment. Remember the senario, "He was good at what he did . . . he achieved success in an unconventional manner . . . they tried to mar his reputation."

In his autobiography, *Through My Eyes*, Dr. Charles D. Kelman explained how he fought to overcome resistance from within the

---

[3]David Seabury, *The Art of Self-Ishness* p. viii.

medical world in his search for a less risky and more effective method of cataract removal. Today, thanks to his persistence, thousands of people see more clearly. Establishment is slow to change, especially when change is being pushed by the new boy on the block.

> *"Progress always involves risk; you can't steal second base and keep your foot on first."*[4]

I was not afraid to take the risk to become a facial surgeon rather than a *general* plastic surgeon. The odds were strongly in my favor because I had defined the problem and prepared to execute the solution.

Christopher Columbus gathered his staff, charted his course and set sail toward the western horizon. Both in planning and executing his expedition, he overcame adversity. Certainly, plastic surgery was being performed in hospitals and offices around the state, but no previous surgeon in Alabama had developed an outpatient facility which specialized exclusively in plastic surgery of the face. This had been my plan since medical school. That is why I chose to direct my training to the head and neck region of the body. Dr. Ellis Porch, years before, had advised me to choose sub-specialization. He saw medicine heading in that direction. Through his experienced eyes, I saw what he saw and set sail toward specialization. As did Columbus, Lindbergh, Akins, and Kelman, I faced some challenges.

The Secret of Success

Coach Paul Bryant won 323 football games, more than any other *major* college coach in history. Why was he more successful than others? On numerous occasions, I heard people, usually reporters, ask Coach Bryant, "What is the secret to your success?" His pat answer was, "If I knew I wouldn't tell YOU." He was a teacher, but he wanted the information to fall upon the ears of his students, not to a reporter who might not tell the story exactly as he intended. Coach had been "burned" many times by the media.

One day he was interviewed on "The Dick Cavett Show." During the show, Cavett asked Coach Bryant "the question." He paused, and

---

[4]Frederick Wilcox, *Motivational Quotes* p. 30.

then said, "Well, I'm going to tell you why I've been successful. I've surrounded myself with people who are smarter than I am and people who are committed to helping me accomplish my goals.

I no longer coach football. I coach people. My assistant coaches do the coaching. I just help them plan what they are going to do. I won't hire anyone who doesn't know more about one aspect of the game (of football) than I know, someone that can do something I don't know how to do or can't do, physically.

"To be successful—to do good things," he went on, "you must surround yourself with good people. If someone in your organization is a weak link, is not doing his job or has a bad attitude, get rid of him. He will pull the rest down. The others will not be able to drag him along and do their jobs effectively. You don't have to motivate good people, nor does the rest of the staff have to waste time correcting their mistakes."

Following Coach Bryant's remarks, I realized, like many business and professional executives, how foolish I had been. I had often hired people with no experience and had to teach them everything I expected them to do. My team was limited as to what it could achieve, because the others only knew what I had taught them. On several occasions, I had hired someone who would come to work for less money rather than an experienced person who could take on responsibility right away—not a smart move when one prepares to sail into rough waters.

Coach Bryant was an offspring of the Knute Rockne football family. He inherited good, professional blood lines. Coach Bryant's coach, when he played at Alabama, was Frank Thomas, who played for and worked with Rockne at Notre Dame before coming to Alabama as head coach.

At the Birmingham Touchdown Club, Coach Bobby Bowden of Florida State University reviewed Knute Rockne's criteria for selecting winners. Fifty-six years ago, Rockne looked for five main qualities in the men he recruited to become members of his team. They were: brains, ambition, dependability, willingness to work, and positive attitude. Coach Bowden added a sixth—enthusiasm. Rockne's "five" have withstood the test of time. Enthusiasm comes from the Greek word "enthias," which means "full of the gods." Combine this with Rockne's five, and you have the characteristics of a winning player (or a staff member) who can be counted on when the chips are down.

Ever since the day I saw Dick Cavett's interview, I have tried to follow Coach Bryant's "secret" to success in putting together my Clinic staff. I've tried to choose good people. It has paid off for me. I know it will for you, too.

In developing my approach to business and building my Clinic, to paraphrase Dale Carnegie, I borrowed ideas from Socrates, Plato, Churchill, Lincoln and Coach Bryant, copied them from Columbus, Anderson, Webster, Berman, Kirklin, Rockne, and Bowden, and followed those of Jesus and Moses. If you don't like their rules, whose would *you* use?

CHAPTER 22

A CASE OF SLANDER

"If you are being kicked from the rear, it may mean that you are up front."[1]

For almost a decade I have conducted continuing medical educational seminars for the American Academy of Facial Plastic and Reconstructive Surgery, Inc. Surgeons from around the world come to Birmingham to share their experiences and to keep current with state of the art techniques in both cosmetic and reconstructive plastic surgery.

The teachers at these seminars share both their good and their not-so-good cases. By doing so, those in attendance benefit from the instructor's unfortunate experiences. Seeing how the "expert" worked through his problem, the student learns how to avoid and/or overcome similar problems should they surface back home.

In like manner, throughout this book, I have taken you into the classroom, the operating room, the football huddle, the locker room and onto the field of battle. Now, I'm going to take you behind the scenes of another kind of "gut check"—an attempted character assassination, one of the greatest personal challenges I've ever faced. The experience was similar to being mugged or raped in a dark alley by a masked bandit who attempted to strip one of his or her dignity.

---

[1]Anonymous, *Seeds To Sow* p. 42.

While searching for ways to respond to these slanderous attacks, I discovered that such assaults are fairly common. I was shocked to learn that character assassinations are used as a tool by competitors in politics, the corporate world, and in the health care professions when they want to bring down someone who is labeled a "threat." Lee Iacocca told the world his story. He inspired me to tell mine.

By 1985, after some twenty-two years of training and work I completed the final edition on the McCollough Facial Surgery Clinic, P.A., fulfilling the dream conceived during my early days in medical school. My practice was going well, my family was happy in our new home and the world tasted good, but the devil was at work.

Coach Bryant said, "the price of victory is high, but so are the rewards."

In my wildest imagination, I never realized that the price one would pay to establish a successful facial plastic surgery practice would be so high. I already knew about the price one had had to pay getting there, but I was not prepared for the price one had to pay afterwards. My family and I were about to face a tragic event. Mark Twain wrote, "It takes your enemy and your friend, working together to hurt you to the heart, the one to slander you and the other to get the news to you."

Even though I should have been flattered when looked upon as such a threat by competitors and detractors, it is still a bitter pill to swallow, one that goes down hard. If, however, as with some treatments, it will ultimately improve the individual's situation, then, maybe, the discomfort associated with the treatment will be worth it. I have to believe that will be the case.

While growing up in Enterprise I never looked upon good fortune, health and happiness as a threat, but I'm learning. "Country boys" are sometimes naive. On the other hand, it doesn't take many stings by a bee to learn that when the critter lites on you, he's not there to pollenate.

Spreaders of Filth

Where did it begin? Why did it occur? What was to be gained? What should I do? I went back to the beginning searching for answers, looking for ways to identify the spreaders of filth.

When the news of my plan to establish my clinic became known within a segment of the medical community, that's when sparks seemed to fly. Was it because we could offer surgery and post-operative care at considerably less cost than existing hospital-based plastic surgery, that we were looked upon as a threat to the stagnant establishment? Today, all medical institutions are moving in this direction.

Did other surgeons performing plastic surgery feel threatened when they heard about my plan? It appeared that they tried to discredit us. I remembered the earlier meeting with two Birmingham general plastic surgeons. I had met with them to see if we could work in the same community on a basis of mutual respect. I thought it was a reasonable plan. I was somewhat shocked when my one-time teachers and friends told me they would attempt to undermine my plan to develop a practice within the community. I was quickly realizing that I had an uphill battle ahead to do what I had planned. I remembered that fourth down play on the goal line in the Orange Bowl.

In a separate meeting that same year, I talked with two other plastic surgeons who I knew less well. One was a gentleman. I have to believe that he has maintained a position of relative neutrality. The other, however, was less open-minded. I'll have to say that they were, at least, up front with their opinions. Some of their colleagues and proteges have not been.

Once some of the obstructionists had been identified and their attitude was made known to me, I was prepared to deal with it. I remembered the words of John Croyle, who had said that once a problem was defined, it was 90% solved. When I had set out to establish my practice, I thought this problem was well-defined. It was, however, far from being solved.

Guerrilla Warfare???

The "country boy" in me assumed that the "game" would be played in the open, by the rules. If that was to be the case, I was willing to accept the challenge. I had been taught to deal with adversity by men who were proven giants in their individual work—my father, my high school coaches, Coach Bryant, Dr. Jack Anderson, Dr. Richard Webster, Drs. James and Julius Hicks, Ellis Taylor, and Dr. Joab Thomas. Each man had shared with me his formula for success and his method of analyzing and predicting human behavior. Following their principles, and trying to provide quality medical care, would offer me the best chance to accomplish my professional goal. With this philosophy as my standard, I had gone to work.

A campaign within the medical community immediately arose which ultimately carried over to the public. The truth about my training and experience in facial plastic surgery and my board-certification was twisted. Apparently, someone was attempting to discredit me, thinking they could hurt my practice, damage my credibility, and ruin my reputation.

I became aware of the campaign when friends and patients informed me of slanderous comments made to them by competing surgeons. As my medical practice grew and I achieved more recognition as an officer in the national facial and cosmetic surgery associations, the slanderous rumors and allegations became more overt, the character assassination campaign to discredit me more vicious.

My children came home from school and said, "Daddy, one of my friends told me they heard you were not *licensed* to do the surgery you do." The implication was that I was doing something illegal.

Confused patients called or came into my office and asked about my training and certification. They had been told by competing surgeons that I was not "board-certified" to do facial surgery, even though my board-certification in otolaryngology certified competence in head and neck plastic surgery. (Not only was I board-certified, I have served as an examiner from the facial plastic academy for other surgeons seeking certification by the American Board of Otolaryngology.) I could see that my competitors' campaign to discredit my credentials and ruin my reputation was gaining momentum.

I wondered if this, too, might be the local implementation of a national campaign spearheaded by some leaders of the national *general* plastic surgery organization (The American Society of Plastic and Reconstructive Surgeons) against surgeons who were not members of their "fraternity" or who were certified by any "Board", other than its own.

Having served as an officer and member of the board of directors of the largest organization of facial or *specialty* plastic surgeons in the world (AAFPRS), I was aware of the expensive public relations campaign initiated by some of the *general* plastic surgeons. In their newsletter, the stated goal was to become the "knowledge broker of plastic surgery." The general plastic surgery society hoped to convince the public that only their members were qualified to perform certain kinds of plastic surgery. One of the largest public relations firms in the world (Hill and Knowlton, Chicago, Illinois) was retained for about $300,000 per year to distribute this edict.

The activities of some of the *general* plastic surgeons and/or their national organization eventually became so blatant, that, as ASPRS anticipated in their 1975 document, the Federal Trade Commission initiated an investigation against one of the general plastic surgery societies for "restraint of trade" and anti-competitive activities. During its investigation, the FTC uncovered another document which appeared to be a master plan, clearly outlining how the *general* plastic surgeons would conduct a "cold war" and use "guerrilla warfare" tactics, similar to those of Vietnam, against fellow physicians and medical organizations they identified as competitors.

Back home in Alabama, in the face of attacks intended to discredit my training and credentials, my practice continued to grow. The plans for a self-contained facility devoted solely to plastic surgery of the face became a reality. Final construction and the interior furnishings of our newly renovated facility were completed in January, 1985.

The News or The Facts

Many lifetime dreams began to materialize during this same period of time. Numerous personal and professional honors were received. I was elected to be president of the American Academy of Facial Plastic and Reconstructive Surgery, Inc. and had been appointed by Governor George Wallace to the Board of Directors of the Alabama Sports Hall of Fame. Good things were happening. In 1981, Former Lt. Governor George McMillan had appointed me to a 5 year term on the Medical Licensure Commission of the State of Alabama. The Commission issues and revolks the licenses of physicians and oversees complaints registered against members of the medical profession. I had been asked to serve on the board of directors of both the Birmingham Area Chamber of Commerce and the Birmingham Better Business Bureau.

The University of Alabama at Birmingham made me a clinical professor in the Department of Surgery and offered to make me Director of the Section of Facial Surgery in the Division of Otolaryngology. Good things continued to happen. My home town had just presented me with an honor of distinction as its All-Time outstanding football player. Dr. Bill Beeson (Indianapolis, Indiana) and I completed a textbook on plastic surgery, *Aesthetic Surgery of the Aging Face* (Mosby). (Dr. Beeson and Dr. Steve Perkins, both of whom did an approved AAFPRS fellowship in facial plastic surgery with me, have been challenged by a general plastic surgeon competitor in Indianapolis).

Back in Alabama, our children were enjoying success in their endeavors. Susan and I were being invited to travel to many interesting places throughout the world to teach other doctors about facial plastic surgery. Life tasted good. The price and rewards of "victory" were all around us.

There is an axiom of Murphy's Law which states "when you think everything is going smoothly, you obviously don't know what is going on." Unfortunately, when we become informed, we wished we hadn't. Too often these days, "the news" is not "the facts." Almost daily, we were informed of a series of vicious rumors that were being circulated around the state of Alabama. I was falsely being accused of all kinds of questionable activities. Imagine the worst possible scenario of rumors that could be assembled. At one time or the other, any or all of that scenario was used against me or some member of my family. A character assassination is the lowest blow which could be delivered to a husband, father, and physician. These tactics have been used in the dirty game of politics and business, but this was my first realization that they are also used against private citizens.

Unlike Iacocca at Ford, I was Chairman of the Board at my clinic. I didn't have to contend with a Henry Ford. There was no one individual who had the power or authority to fire me, but a number of other similarities did exist. He was also looked upon as a threat by an adversary.

On February 12, 1986, Iacocca was fired from the Statue of Liberty Restoration Committee by Interior Secretary Donald Hodell. Iacocca had helped raise over 250 million dollars for a "face-lift" for the Statue and also headed up a committee who was overseeing the work. A "conflict of interest" it was called. Personally, I think it stinks. He has become a hero. His book is the third best seller of all time, behind *Gone With the Wind* and *Jonathon Livingston Seagull*. The proceeds of his book *Iacocca* are being donated to the Joslin Diabetes Center in Boston, and I doubt if he received a salary for his work on the Statue of Liberty project.

In *Ben Hur,* Lew Wallace wrote: "A man is never so on trial as in the moment of excessive good fortune."

From my own experiences I have learned that "gutless" opponents play a different game—they hit below the belt. Like mice, they sneak out from their holes and spread their filth. Traps are made for mice and fools. Now, the problem was defined. The solution became more apparent.

Slander and The Law

Most people who spread untrue rumors of a slanderous nature do not realize the risk they take; for in doing so in the state of Alabama, they are violating the law.

I asked my good friend and legal counsel, Ed Hardin, to search Alabama law with regard to the repeating of slander. I was somewhat surprised at his response, and I think most of the readers of this book will be, too.

The question was:

Is "one who repeats a rumor or remark that is slanderous per se, even though that person acknowledges that the statement is repeated from another source, liable for slander?

The answer was:

"Yes, one who repeats a defamatory statement (slander per se) made by someone else is considered to have published it, and is liable as if he were the first person to make the statement. This is true even if he indicates that he does not believe the statement to be true."

Loose talk can be dangerous; particularly when it is untrue and is damaging to the character and reputation of the victim. The Alabama Code (of law) is clear on this matter. It provides, in part that, ". . . one who repeats or otherwise republishes defamatory matter is subject to liability as if he had originally published it," and treats the speaker of a slanderous remark as liable, if he "accompanies the slander with a statement that it is a rumor only or designates the name of the author or original publisher." This rule is applicable although the listener may have already heard similar statements from other sources.

When the slanderous rumors began to reflect on our children,

Susan and I felt we could no longer sit idly by and simply hope the rumors would go away. They seemed to become more widespread and more vicious with each passing month, often being repeated aloud in large groups of people as though there were a concerted effort to disseminate them quickly and widely. I was shocked to learn what some people will believe. Adversaries were pouring on the fuel while the wheels of the rumor mill were turning. It seemed that anyone who ever had an ax to grind relished in the thought that just maybe they had found something to use against my family and me.

When a private investigator identified that the rumors seemed to be flourishing within the medical community, we decided the first step would be to try to alert the local physicians of the problem and to serve notice to the guilty parties that they had gone too far with their attempted character assassination. After appropriate consultation, a letter was sent to the physician community asking for the help of those who were not involved. We considered sending a similar letter to beauty shops, figure skating clubs, travel agencies and country clubs. The letter was a risky move, sure to raise some eyebrows and draw criticism. It gave people something else to discuss.

Retrospectively, maybe we overreacted. My family and I had been cut deeply. We were bleeding to death. The first thing to do, we decided, was to try to stop the bleeding, then we could worry about the associated complications.

The letter seemed to achieve much of the desired effect. A number of our friends stepped forward to help us. I received calls and letters confirming the slanderous statements and their authors. We also received other types of communications. One careless sender of an obscene letter used a registered postage meter from an architectural office in our business community.

Character assassinations are not only immoral and unethical, but are also illegal. The law, we learned, provides for protection against such conduct.

According to Shakespeare, who is credited for penning the word "assassination," rumor is based upon "surmises, jealousies and conjectures."

Rumor, I learned, is also a tool used to harm by those who feel threatened and don't have the guts to face a "threat" head on—snipers hiding in trees fire bullets at targets they fear to challenge face to face—social and professional terrorism.

I fully expected resistance while trying to achieve my professional goals, but I honestly never expected to face unfounded assaults upon my manhood, morals, and ethics by people whose only intent was to harm. I must admit that when this attempted character assassination was revealed to me, I was devastated. What had I done, or not done, to deserve this? Was this part of the price of victory? I began to search for answers and to try to identify who was responsible. I fought back in the only way I knew—head on. I remember hearing someone say, "If it walks like a duck and quacks like a duck, there is a good chance that it is a duck."

With this premise in mind, and with the help of our friends and private investigators, we began to zero in on *some* of the "ducks" . . . and "mice" spreading their filth. Once we had them in our sights we had a choice to make. Do we blast them with a slander suit or not? I felt like the solution to my dilemma must have been worked out by some great man who faced a similar predicament.

I came across an incident described by Charles Lindbergh, the great American aviator, during World War II.[2] He was flying a security mission over one of the small, but strategic, Pacific Islands, in search of "targets of opportunity," when he came upon a man on the beach. From the man's posture and stride, Lindbergh was convinced that he must be an enemy officer, possibly a general. The man was alone and obviously unarmed as though he had been separated from his troops. He was a sitting duck for an ace like Lindbergh.

As he circled and guided his aircraft on target for the kill, Lindbergh placed his finger on the trigger of the plane's machine gun. In an instant, he came face to face with life, and death. He held the Japanese officer's life in his hand. There they were, just the two of them, both realizing the power one had over the other. Rarely do the powerful submit to the powerless.

Lindbergh owed humanity one. Before the war, he had been rescued from disaster by a Japanese sailing vessel. His finger froze on the trigger, then he gently removed it completely, and the plane passed over the man on the beach as he walked into the jungle, and disappeared.

He could have destroyed his enemy. They were at war. It would have been the "proper" thing to do, under the circumstances, but Lindbergh chose to live and let live.

When the identities of my enemies and their emissaries were re-

---

[2]Charles H. Lindbergh, *Autobiography of Values* (Jovanovich, Schiff).

vealed, I concluded that *this time* we would not use the "bullets" we had at our disposal. I would give them one more chance. I spurned the trigger and decided to soar on past. The bullets were saved for another day.

"My Good Name"

Former Alabama Governor "Big Jim" Folsom was the victim of much criticism. He handled it by the following philosophy:

> *"When your enemies sling mud, don't smear it in, just let it dry and it brushes off easily without leaving a mark."*

When I am confronted with a difficult situation, I usually try to draw upon past experiences and the wisdom of great men.

Shakespeare wrote, "who steals my purse steals trash; . . . But he that filches from me *my good name* robs me of that which not enriches him, and makes me poor indeed."

I realized that no one could rob from me "my good name" unless I allowed it to happen.

In the face of his first international humiliation, Iacocca didn't roll over and play dead. He channeled his energies into his work at Chrysler and brought a dying corporation back from the grave. He also may emerge as the Statue of Liberty's "first gentleman."

Coach Bryant dealt with the assault upon his character by blasting those who falsely accused him of "fixing" the 1964 Alabama vs. Georgia football game.

One difference between mine and the two previous situations is that from the beginning they knew who their detractors were. The similarity, however, is that each profited from his gut-check. As I analyzed my problem, I realized that it would be necessary to draw upon wisdom from the giants of the present and the past.

Difficulties either make us *bitter* or *better*. Like the ones with which I have been faced in the past, this difficulty is being used in like manner—to help make me a better person. The rumormongers may have done me much more good than harm. The disillusioned Don Quixote spent the wanning years of his life pursuing "The Impossible Dream," fighting windmills. Windmills are not threats. They remain in one place and simply go 'round and 'round until they decay.

Had "The Man From La Mancha" realized this fact, he could have quickly and surely won that battle by ignoring them and moving forward to more noble goals.

The Delegation of Vengeance

Could the slander dilemma be just another "gut check"? They continue to surface throughout life. This goal line shall be crossed without question. My team will "walk in." The winners will be my children, my wife, and my parents, and all those who have instilled their trust and confidence in me along the way. In the end, there will be no place for doubt. This time, there will be no chance for anyone to shade the truth in the record book of life's game.

For thousands of years, rumors have been used against men and women who are trying to accomplish a goal devious minds oppose.

When Nehemiah was rebuilding the great wall around Jerusalem, a malicious rumor was circulated accusing him of fraudulent motives and methods. His adversaries were attempting to discredit him and to keep him from achieving his goal by turning public opinion against him. Through a hired emissary they tried to drive him into seclusion and away from his objective.

> *"They hired him (the emissary) to frighten me (Nehemiah) . . . So that they could ruin my reputation and humiliate me."*[3]

Nehemiah knew he was on the side of right. With God's help, the great wall of Jerusalem was rebuilt. His enemies lost face, maybe more.

Once again, I found the answer to a dilemma by drawing upon the wisdom of a giant, proving that there are no new problems, just new characters, dates, and places. The struggle between good and evil is as old as time itself. The fate of each is predictable.

Irresponsible people will ultimately be brought to justice. Truth will prevail. One day, before our Creator, each human being will have to account for his actions and deeds. The jury will be fair, but stern.

---

[3]*Good News Bible,* Nehemiah 6:13.

*"The divine wrath is slow . . . in vengeance, but it makes
up for its tardiness by the severity of the punishment"*[4]

I decided to go on about my work while the mice play in their filth.
They'll come out of their holes again. That's their nature. You'll see
what I mean. Next time the "man on the beach" might not be so
lucky.

It Ain't Over

What we do with our life is a matter of choice. Will the choice be
excellence, mediocrity, or oblivion? This is a question each of us has
to answer.

In his song, "The Gambler," Kenny Rogers deals us "an ace." The
ballad suggests that in life's game each of us is dealt a hand of cards.
Each player decides how his hand is to be played. "Every hand's a
winner and every hand's a loser." The cards dealt to us only provide
a *chance* in life's game. The "secret to survival" depends upon making the right *choices*—"knowing what to throw away and knowing
what to keep." The right choices are made by acquiring wisdom from
those wiser than us.

When the time comes for a show-down each player analyzes his
strengths and weaknesses, then makes a decision to hold or fold. The
great players win more than they lose, however, "The Gambler" advises us not to total the score too soon. "There'll be time enough for
counting when the dealings done."

I have not yet done everything I want, nor need to do. I'm not yet
ready to total the score. Yogi Berra said, "It ain't over, 'til it's over.' "
This game "ain't" over—there's more dealing to be done.

A Critic Is An Asset

I believe that I have been exposed to great people (and devious
people) so that I could learn to handle adversity. Throughout life, we
are confronted with "gut-checks." The great philosopher, Horace,
said, "adversity has the effect of eliciting talents, which in prosper-

---

[4]Valerius Maximus, *10,000 Jokes* (Copeland), p. 670.

ous times would have lain dormant." The lowly mongoose is at his best when challenged by the venomous cobra.

I have learned that on the tail of every achievement lies an adversity. We can expect to face that reality until "the dealing's done." It is also necessary, however, to remember that on the tail of every adversity lies an opportunity for further achievement.

A prominent businessman, politician and member of the social register said the attacks upon my family and me arose from maintaining "too high of a profile" in this community and recommended I change that. Three months later, I received a promotional brochure espousing the accomplishments of his son who was seeking support for an elected political office. I realized then that whether or not one is maintaining "too high a profile" depends upon who's doing the evaluating.

Andrew Carnegie once said, "As I grow older, I pay less attention to what men say. I just watch what they do." Deeds transcend debates. I have yet to campaign for public office. Any notoriety I have received is a result of work in the classroom, athletic arena, operating room, or as a teacher.

Should we be concerned about criticism dealt by any narrowminded, self-anointed segment of society which feels that the rest of us should stay "in our place" until we have paid our dues? Attempts to discredit the efforts of those of us who have not been "knighted" goes against the "pull yourself up by the bootstraps" philosophy that I have been taught.

On the evening of February 22, 1986, I participated in my first Alabama Sports Hall of Fame induction ceremony as a member of the Board of Directors. Under the chairmanship of Larry Striplin we inducted six outstanding Alabamians into the Sports Hall of Fame: Sam Perry, Bill Lee, Bobby Marlow, Bobby Bowden, Terry Beasley, and Kenny Stabler. None of these men reached the pinnacle in athletics by trying to maintain a low profile or waiting on the approval of others. They went about their activities with zest, enthusiasm, and commitment. In doing so, they became the best they could be. That is why their names become an indelible record in the museum which honors great Alabama sportsmen.

Low profiles, I believe, are for those who have something to hide, or are gutless. I have concluded that some individuals who enjoy high profiles usually want everyone *else* to maintain a low one.

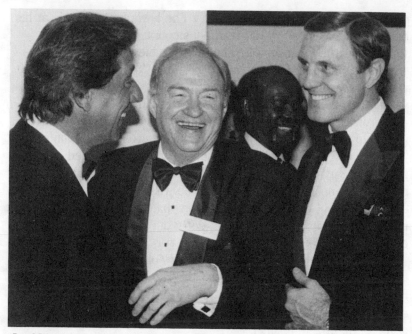

*Joe Namath, Larry Striplin, and Gaylon McCollough at the 1986
Alabama Sports Hall of Fame induction ceremonies.*

As a young man I accepted Winston Churchill's challenge when he
advised,

> *"Come on now all you young men all over the world. . .
> Don't be content with things as they are. . . Don't take no
> for an answer, never submit to failure. Do not be fobbed off
> with mere personal success or acceptance. You (will) make
> all kinds of mistakes; but as long as you are generous and
> true, and also fierce, you cannot hurt the world or even se-
> riously distress her. . . she is made to be wooed and won by
> youth."[5]*

Churchill, a wise man, is one of my heroes. His courage helped
save Britain in the darkest days She ever witnessed.

Another bit of wisdom was given to me by Dr. Dennis Pappas. An

---

[5]Bartlett, *While England Slept* p. 920.

older man who had helped Pappas build The Lanterns (his beautiful home) said to him, "Doc, never apologize for being successful."

When he heard about the attempts to discredit me, another friend, Dr. Milton Rubin, sent me the following piece of advice: "You will be criticized if there is any force whatsoever to your personality. There is just one way to avoid criticism: Never do anything, never amount to anything. Get your head above the crowd and the jealous will notice and criticize you. Therefore, criticism is a sign that your life has vitality."

After reflecting upon these words, I realize that maybe I have been able to become a better facial surgeon because some of my competitors and detractors have made it even a greater challenge. I tend to thrive upon being backed into a corner. Tell me I can't and I'll try to show you I can. I will not apologize for doing so. If the second wave of social and professional terrorism comes, I shall be better prepared. Self-analysis, self-esteem, and self-control are the keys to dealing with assaults. When we are in control, destiny is a matter of choice.

The Country In Me

Mark Twain once said, "In Boston they ask, How much does he know? In New York, How much is he worth? In Philadelphia, Who were his parents?"

Sometimes, *they* don't ask anything, *they* simply try to undermine and control. *They* often underestimate the power of commitment and the strength of the desire to succeed. The *Post* underestimated Coach Bryant, Ford underestimated Iacocca. The British underestimated the early American Colonies. Sanballat underestimated Nehemiah, and Goliath underestimated David.

I believe that *what we are* and *what we intend to do* is more important than where we live, who our ancestors were, to which social club set we belong, or which diploma hangs on our wall. Fools get hung up on family trees. Birth is simply the beginning. There's more, much, much more afterwards. Good blood lines are a great start. Blood, however, only serves as the carrier of the oxygen that nourishes the brain. What we do with our genetic gift is another matter. Sir T. Overbury said, "The man who has not anything to boast about but his illustrious ancestors, is like a potato—the only thing belonging to him is under ground."[6]

Some people, I believe, get their priorities and objectives confused. They strive to be accepted by society. They believe that they must speak a certain way, wear the approved attire, drive the appropriate automobile, belong to a certain country club, and socialize with the right people in order to be acceptable. This philosophy develops clones, carbon copies of the prototype developed by those who control the social register. It inhibits new ideas, growth and progress. Thank God Christopher Columbus, Thomas Jefferson, Abe Lincoln, Winston Churchill, Douglas MacArthur, and Thomas Edison weren't clones. These men were not afraid to dream, scheme, and act. They transcended mediocrity. Leaders generally do.

We live in a society that is blessed with procedural behavior. Too often, the process of living overshadows the purpose of our existence.

In his address to the 1986 Alabama Sports Hall of Fame breakfast, Tom Skinner told the story about how he went into a basketball game with the right attitude and preparation. In his desire to do all the appropriate things, he lost perspective of his objective. He enthusiastically intercepted a pass and charged toward the goal, being careful not to break any of the rules or draw a foul. He jumped off the correct foot, used the proper hand, laid the ball into the basket with precision, grace, and style, and scored two points—for the *opposing* team. He became so obsessed with doing things right that he lost perspective. He got his priorities mixed up. The process was right. The goal and direction were wrong.

Procedural behavior must not prevent one from pursuing noble goals. As long as the goal and direction is moral and right, the method matters little.

Why shouldn't one attempt to improve himself? Is anything wrong with trying to be the best that he can be with the cards life has dealt to him? Isn't that the American way?

A "high profile," I guess, means committing one's time, energies, and resources to try to better himself, his cause, his profession, his community, his family, and his school—to reinvest what he has learned so that others might have the same chance he did.

---

[6]*Treasury of Familiar Quotations* p. 9.

If that sounds corny, so be it. I live by that philosophy! I guess that's just the country in me. I am who I am. After all, I did come from a small town in south Alabama. I grew up admiring *real* people—people who liked you for *what* you are; people who take pride in their work and feel good about themselves when they have successfully completed a task; people who were not afraid to dream and talk about ideas and goals rather than about other people's faults; people who realize that a world exists beyond the city limits of their own community.

Little minds need to dwell in little places, think little thoughts, and do little things, but I do not intend to change my "profile" to conform to the narrow-minded standards of my critics. I believe that I have been blessed with some talents and abilities and that it is my responsibility to do something with them.

I am not yet finished with what I want to do for my family, my profession, my teachers and friends, my community, or for myself. If I want to avoid criticism I could choose to "do nothing, say nothing, and be nothing." That kind of existence would be synonymous with retirement or death and I'm not yet prepared to voluntarily accept either. Not yet.

Looking back at the problem and the solution, if I could be given a second chance, I don't think I would alter my plan, my goals, or my methods. Knowing I would face an attempted character assassination, I would do it all again. Having now survived another kind of "gut-check," I could advise any person who has a dream to go for it. Stay on the side of right and let the mice play. In the end, they may be of more help than harm.

> "... *He that wrestles with us strengthens*
> *our nerves and sharpens our skills.*
> *Our antagonists is our helper.* . ."[7]

---

[7]Burk, *Treasury of Familiar Quotations* p. 78.

CHAPTER 23

ANATOMY OF AN INDIVIDUALIST

"Experience is a hard teacher because she gives the test first, the lesson afterwards"[1]

One of my main goals throughout life has been to reverse this statement. By studying the experiences of others, it is possible to acquire some of their wisdom *before* you take your test—a much easier and more direct route than trial and error. I have tried to follow behind those with "loaded wagons." When something falls out, I want to be there to pick it up.

Before we can incorporate the teachings of great and experienced people into our own lives, however, we must first find out who we are (self-analysis). A popular song ("The Greatest Love Of All") tells us that, first, we must learn to love ourselves (self-esteem).

I have concluded that I have been first, and always, an individualist. During my boyhood days, I enjoyed the solitude of fishing on the river bank, hunting in the woods, and riding my horse along the dirt roads and fields of southeastern Alabama. Those times allowed me to analyze myself, gave me the opportunity to explore my dreams and decide who and what I wanted to become.

---

[1]Vernon Law, *Friends* (Kaplans).

During my years as an athlete, I learned how to function as a team player, and to fight for what I believe to be right and moral and for what I believed to be in the best interest of my family, my friends, and my cause.

I am driven to ask How and Why and dream of how things might be instead of accepting things as they are. I attempt to build upon a positive self-esteem through the accomplishment of goals I have set for myself. I am happiest when seeking opportunity, not security. I look for the challenges in life and believe in the good and the positive. I dream and plan, then work while others play in order to achieve my goals. I detest negative thoughts, but try to be realistic; look for the hidden flaw and try to have an alternate plan so that I am in control of my own destiny. From the shoulders of some of the giants I have credited, I am looking toward the future, searching for their secrets of self-fulfillment. At the same time I am pursuing an even better way of life. If my experiences can serve as a lesson to help one other person better himself, then my efforts have been worthwhile. That is the responsibility of a teacher. It is the purpose of this book.

Only A Beginning

The Bible tells us "this too shall pass." Good or bad, no condition is permanent on life's roller coaster. The bad times afford a man the opportunity to examine his convictions.

David Mallet advised "Who hath not known ill fortune, never knew himself, or his own virtue."

I have learned from the men and women who were and are my teachers. By example, they showed us that if we outworked our adversaries we could outlast our critics. As long as one has the confidence of his family, friends, and business associates, little else matters. I have chosen to continue in the pursuit of excellence, and to draw upon the wisdom of great men and women, cognizant of the fact that ill-wishers would have me fail. That is their choice.

Public opinion alone must not dictate an individual's actions. Someone once said "The man who trims himself to suit everybody will soon whittle himself away."[2]

Throughout history, great people have taken calculated risks in or-

---

[2]Anonymous, *Seeds To Sow* p. 23.

der to accomplish their goals. In the end, many of their scoffers have been the benefactors. Does one wait for a sign of approval before stepping toward his destiny? It has been written that "He who must wait on [the approval of] others can start when *they* [others] are ready, he who goes alone can begin immediately."[3] I've only been at this thing called life for 43 years, only a beginning: I can't wait to see what my next 43 will produce. Susan and I might open up a "branch office," an international cosmetic surgery clinic in some exotic resort area, maybe the Carribean or even Monte Carlo. What about a floating cosmetic surgery hospital? Before the rumors fly, we aren't leaving Birmingham; however, it might be fun to expand our horizons. I might even try my hand at politics in a few years. It "ain't" over. Not yet.

There are things yet to do, problems yet to solve, choices yet to make.

---

[3]*Seeds to Sow.*

Part V

A LOOK AT MEDICINE AND THE LAW

CHAPTER 24

AMERICA AWAITS THE VERDICT

From my vantage point, I can see that Americans will face some serious problems in the years ahead. We desperately need leaders to step forward from both the health care professions and the private sector. A new game plan must be developed. A winning team must be fielded, based upon knowledge, courage, and wisdom.

Because the public is a participant, it too needs to be informed of some of the variables which will determine the future of medicine. The time has come to become partners in health. Working together, the problems can be solved. We have been given the tools and abilities to control our own destiny.

Doctors must get their act together because a number of problems face the medical profession. How the physician community deals with them will determine the manner in which the public will receive medical care and what the medical profession will become within the next quarter of a century.

In the book, *Doing Better and Feeling Worse,* some of the dilemmas facing health care in the United States are concisely stated. Physicians have been accused of a conspiracy of silence; however, some of the problems the profession faces, from within and without, shall be discussed openly and honestly. The public needs to know. The public is part of the new team.

During the past 25 years, there has been increasing specialization in medicine, so that by 1980, more that 70 percent of all American physicians were specialists.

There is now one medical doctor for every 645 people. With increased enrollment in medical schools, the number of doctors is increasing at an even more dramatic rate. According to the capitalistic philosophy, supply follows demand. Although some insiders who fear competition have argued that we are training too many doctors, anyone who has had difficulty obtaining treatment in the face of illness or who waits two or three hours to see his or her doctor would have a difficult time accepting an argument that we have too many doctors. Maybe today we need more family physicians and fewer sub-specialists. Those who control the numbers game may not be able to keep the lid on much longer. The market place should decide the issue.

Certain conditions, once considered criminal behavior, are now categorized as medical conditions. Alcoholism, drug addiction and psychopathic behavior now fall under the classification of medical or psychiatric disorders. The burden of responsibility has been shifted from the individual to society, from the jail cell to the hospital.

Who is to blame? This trend may have developed because of the difficulty political leaders have had in dealing with criminal behavior for fear of having a liberal-thinking Supreme Court overturn their decisions. The laws relative to punishment and the overcrowding of prisons may open doors for blaming irresponsible behavior on medical conditions rather than on environmental conditions. Today, there are more hospital beds than prison cells. [1] Maybe some of the dollars spent on such "health care" would better be spent on increasing the salaries and prestige of those who enforce our laws and less on the criminals. We should be more concerned about the rights of the victim, and less concerned about the rights of the criminals.

On the other hand, hospitals, medical organizations, and practitioners have marketed the health care business and the public has bought it. Good health and well-being have become commodities that every American feels someone owes him.

During my facial plastic surgery training, I worked other jobs to help support my family. For a while, I was the Medical Director for a

---

[1] *Feeling Better, Doing Worse.*

large nursing home corporation. In those days, I witnessed families taking advantage of the system. Because the government-sponsored programs allowed it, families would help their elderly parent dispose of his or her possessions in order to become eligible for the Medicaid program. They didn't do anything illegal, but they did take advantage of the government's attempt to care for those who truly were in need. This type of premeditated poverty is done by choice and for economic benefit. A partially socialistic system loaded down with government funded programs invites abuse by the few who know how to play the game.

In the recent past, Congress has granted the "right" of good health by the implementation of numerous reimbursement programs. No matter how hard we try, it is impossible to legislate pride, honesty, and responsibility. Americans can "darn" some of the holes in our health care problem with reason.

A New Partner

The health care problem has been a complex one which involves three parties: the medical profession, the government, and the patient himself. The new health care team for the elderly and under privileged becomes "doctor-government-patient." Notice that the government now occupies a position between the doctor and the patient.

The physician of the 1980's spends almost as much of his time with bureaucratic paperwork, putting out professional "brush fires," and practicing defensive medicines as he does in actual patient care. Extensive records are necessary in order to defend expensive law suits. Today, every new patient represents a potential malpractice law suit. Record keeping has become as important as any other facet of health care. Organized seminars are given to teach proper techniques in record keeping. In an era where health has become a precious commodity, the process of delivery is becoming more complex.

Dr. James Hicks often said that the most important aspect of helping a patient get well is to get them with their doctor. Because of the red tape and the current tort laws, the judicial system and legal profession are becoming important players. The new health care "team" includes the doctor, the government, the patient, the lawyer, and the courts.

Americans have come to expect much from their doctors and we from ourselves. Higher expectations often result in higher achievements, but let us not lose perspective. The printing on the coveted degree states "physician" not "magician." Doctors are human beings who have gone to school a few more years and learned some of the healing art, but the human element and its limitations must never be overlooked.

A physician's performance in caring for his patients is limited to some degree by the information available to him at the time of decision. The patient's general condition, attitude toward illness or wellness and the body's ability to ward off disease while responding to treatment are key factors often overlooked by a society who believes that 20th century medicine can fix or replace anything.

Today's physician must be informed about all kinds of problems. He is asked to advise patients on everything from sagging anatomies to sleep and learning disorders. He must, however, be aware of the fact that his patients, too, are better informed about the factors influencing both illness and wellness than ever before.

A New Crisis

There are ever increasing concerns in health care over rights rather than privileges.[2] The public has higher than ever expectations about what the medical profession ought to be able to accomplish and to prevent. Some are warranted, some not. The rapidly escalating numbers of malpractice suits seem to be not only a reaction to errors and abuses committed by some physicians, but a reflection of how the medical profession is being held *personally* responsible for things often beyond its control. Many of these unfortunate events were once considered scientific and technological uncertainties or "acts of God." In today's society, we have come to the belief that someone must accept the blame for any event. No doubt there are situations in which someone should, but not to the extent many Americans have come to expect.

Today, the ease at which a plaintiff can file a lawsuit in some states and the lucrative potential financial awards which can be realized by attorneys (who often get 50 per cent of the amount of "damages"

---

[2]*Ibid.*

awarded a plaintiff by a jury) compose a large part of the problem. It is not uncommon to see multimillion dollar awards given by juries. If a jury awarded $5 million to an injured party, his attorney might get $2.5 million the jury thought they were awarding to the person in need. Then the "expenses" incurred in preparing the case for trial are deducted from the plaintiff's half. In the end, who is the big winner? We must bring some sanity to this "malpractice crises" by educating prospective jurors and through legislative efforts. The laws which allow so many unwarranted suits to be filed can and must be changed. No one is denying that wrongdoing exists in some cases. In such cases, the patient should be cared for, but is it right for anyone to "get rich" over an unfortunate occurrence? Multimillion dollar awards are becoming too common. The attorney who lands such a case finds the goose capable of laying golden eggs. No wonder the lawyer's heart is in the closing argument, pleading that the jury be merciful. Skilled professionals should be well paid for their training, knowledge and experience, but that is not the issue. What, then, is the issue?

Because of gigantic awards, in some states physician's malpractice insurance premiums have been increasing at the rate of 200 percent per year. Some specialists in America pay as much as $90,000 per year for insurance, if they can get it, just so they can continue to practice.

Many doctors are electing to give up "risky" procedures. Delivering babies, an event that for thousands of years occurred without the presence of a trained professional, has been designated as one of the most risky procedures performed by doctors. Those who still deliver babies have been placed by insurance companies into the *highest* risk category to be insured—higher than cardiac surgeons or neurosurgeons. Doctors who continue to deliver babies are forced to pay exorbitant insurance premiums or stop practicing. I heard a member of the Alabama State Legislature say on the Public Broadcasting System that no longer would a single doctor practicing between Eufaula, Alabama and Montgomery, Alabama (almost a 100 mile span) dare deliver a baby.

Birth defects of any kind, even those which existed before doctors assisted with most deliveries, are being blamed on the doctors who deliver today's defective baby. Is it truly the *doctor's* fault that the baby was defective? Was it malpractice or an accident of nature? The decision is usually left to the court.

Malpractice: A Misnomer

What exactly is meant by "malpractice"? A close examination of the facts reveals that the term is often used incorrectly. *Black's Law Dictionary* defines "malpractice" as "any professional misconduct, unreasonable lack of skill or fidelity in professional or fiduciary duties, evil practice, or illegal or immoral conduct." When applied to physicians it generally implies "professional misconduct toward a patient which is considered reprehensible either because it is immoral in itself or because it is contrary to law or is expressly forbidden by law."

The term has been used to mean, more specifically, "bad, wrong, or injudicious treatment of a patient, professionally and in respect to the particular disease or injury, resulting in injury, unnecessary suffering, or death to the patient, *and proceeding from ignorance, carelessness, want of proper professional skill, disregard of established rules or principles, neglect or a malicious or criminal intent.*"

These are strong allegations. A segment of the legal profession seems to believe that the meaning of "malpractice" should be bent to imply that a physician or a medical provider ought to be held responsible for anything and everything that happens, even though such events may be beyond his control. The doctor is considered the "captain of the ship." Could the malpractice crisis be the event that overloads the ship, or fleet, taking the captains down, too?

We have entered an era of believing that man is accountable to man, even for events previously considered to be "acts of God."

In the March 7th edition of the *Birmingham News*, the problem of increasing lawsuits was reviewed. The dilemma not only involves the medical field, but has spilled over into other segments of society. A letter to the editor from Don Carmichael, Jr. stated that:

—"In one state, an insurance company was ordered to pay $260,000 plus $1,000 per month to a plaintiff who was injured when he fell through a skylight while burglarizing a school.

—One jury ordered Sears to pay an obese man with a heart condition $1.8 million after he had a heart attack while starting a Sears lawn mower."

These stories sound almost too ridiculous to be true.

I read about a case in which a woman had a "tummy tuck" in order to remove a fold of loose skin in her abdomen. Following the surgery, she claimed that her "belly button" was off center. The jury awarded her and her attorneys a *large* sum of money. It seems that the figure was around $700,000.

The public bears the burden of the cost of defending lawsuits and excessive verdicts. The businessman passes on the costs of liability insurance to the consumer. Don Carmichael also asked us to consider the following:

— "About $5.00 of a $25.00 stepladder goes to cover insurance premiums.

— As much as 30% of the cost of some airplanes goes to the liability premiums paid by the manufacturer.

— Football helmets cost $70 to $80 each. About $30 of that goes to liability insurance premiums."

Attempts are being made to correct some of the problems within our legal system. Many pragmatic attorneys recognize the seriousness of the dilemma and support tort reform. The pendulum has swung too far. Reasonable professionals recognize that something must be done. It will be an uphill battle, but one that can be won if Americans choose to do it.

When he practiced law in Springfield, Illinois, it was a common thing for Abraham Lincoln to discourage unnecessary lawsuits, and he was continually sacrificing opportunities to make money.

> *One man who asked him to bring suit for $2.50 against a debtor would not be put off in his passion for revenge.* (A far cry from the colossal awards sought by some of today's plaintiffs.) *His counsel, Lincoln, therefore, gravely demanded $10.00 as a retainer. Half of this he gave to the poor defendant, who, therefore, confessed judgment and paid the $2.50 to his creditor. Thus, the suit was ended to the entire satisfaction of the angry creditor.*[3]

Several years ago, I stopped accepting cases in which people obtained facial scarring from an accident when litigation was involved. Patients would often be referred to us by their attorney. After several office visits counseling with the patient, preparing numerous reports for their attorneys, followed by depositions and court appearances as an "expert witness," we found that only about 20 per cent of the pa-

---

[3]Fuller, *Anecdotes* p. 455.

tients had surgical correction of their scars once the cash settlement had been made by the defendant or by his insurance company. The money seemed to ease the pain and suffering alleged in the plaintiff attorney's legal documents. The appearance of the permanent scar appeared to be much more tolerable. I was beginning to feel like a hired witness rather than a surgeon. I found that, in my clinic, the best policy was to reserve consultations for patients who desired surgical correction *after* the case had been settled. This has worked well for us.

At the time of this writing, I've not yet been in the courtroom as a defendant. The odds are not in my favor. My time will come. The title on my diploma reads "Doctor of Medicine."

An Air of Mystique

Some of the malpractice problem may lie in the belief that there seems to be an air of mystique surrounding the medical profession.

At the conclusion of a long eulogy the speaker proclaimed to a brother physician, "What a genius you are!"

"A genius!" he replied. "For 37 years I've practiced medicine 14 hours a day, and now they call me a genius."[4]

This mystique is not only spontaneously inferred upon doctors and surgeons by the public, but, too often, it is also cultivated by some groups of physicians who claim that they command knowledge and skills too sophisticated to be freely and fully shared with lay persons, or with some of their medical colleagues. This type of arrogance makes the profession an easy target for vultures. Physicians must first be realistic about the M.D. degree and what "board-certification" really means. The public can be misled. Advertising campaigns by physician groups tend to promote higher expectations on the part of the public and lead to confusion. Interspecialty conflicts pit one physician against another. An aggrieved plaintiff and his attorney then take the "cold war" into the courtrooms. Patients are suing their doctors, doctors in turn are suing their patients, and doctors are suing each other. In either case, the lawyers always win.

---

[4]Edmund Fuller, *2500 Anecdotes for All Occasions,* Arenel Books, 190 p. 240.

I often wonder how much legal malpractice would be uncovered if each trial was scrutinized as closely as are the records of doctors and hospitals. Hungry lawyers could have a field day suing each other. If a doctor loses a case of malpractice, was his own attorney negligent? Did his counsel overlook an important document, fail to call the right witness, ask the right questions, follow the best procedure or raise the appropriate objection? Should the public expect any less from the legal profession than it has come to expect from physicians?

While in Palm Beach, Florida, during the spring meeting of the AAFPRS, I saw numerous television commercials in which plaintiff attorneys were asking anyone who was unhappy with any type of medical treatment, anyone who had sustained an injury or had been involved in an accident to contact the attorney's office and consider filing a lawsuit. Similar commercials are aired on Birmingham television. Soon we may see attorneys asking clients of other attorneys who have lost a case in court or who were unhappy with the amount of money they received (even if they won the case) to consult their office and see if they were properly represented. He who lives by the sword. . . .

One of the criteria necessary to get a medical malpractice case before a jury is to have another physician testify that the physician being sued did not follow an arbitrary "standard of care." Certainly with the abundance of attorneys, (one for every 60 people in New York City) one can find lawyers who would be anxious to review trial cases and determine if standards were followed by the attorneys representing the losing side.

What about an income tax return? I'm sure some witch-hunting accountant could find an error of omission on a return prepared by another accountant.

In the courtroom, plaintiffs and defendants deserve no less skill and professionalism than they do elsewhere. Often times, the stakes are high. The client's business, home, reputation, or even his life, may be on the line. Are Americans willing to accept one set of standards for the medical profession and another for the legal profession?

When the average attorney's own legal malpractice insurance premium reaches the $90,000 mark, the legal profession will be seeking tort reform from their colleagues who generally control legislatures.

Blame for today's state of affairs must be shared by each of the involved parties—doctors, lawyers, insurance companies, and greedy plaintiffs hoping for a windfall. The responsibility of putting malpractice claims into perspective must be shared by judges and jurors. Who shall take the lead?

Even during this period when medicine and the medical profession are being subjected to increased scrutiny, criticism, and escalating malpractice claims, each year medical schools around the U.S., on the average, have more than three persons apply for each medical school place available to first year students.[5]

The desire of young people to become physicians speaks well for the continued high esteem to which physicians are held by most of the public. That "esteem" is coveted. It must be earned and preserved.

The condition of American medicine is serious, but it can recover providing it receives the proper care. Recovery is dependent upon all parties doing what must be done, even though it may be a bitter pill to swallow.

The Health We Deserve

Today, good health seems to be best achieved through teamwork. The physician is only one member of that team. The patient is another. Being realistic, we Americans generally have the health we deserve.

Until about 50 years ago the American public placed the greatest emphasis upon the obligations of the individual towards society. That's how we became a great nation. Now, however, the emphasis is increasingly placed upon the obligation of society towards the individual. This attitude is a cancer eating away at our very existence.

Many experts believe that "if cigarette smoking were to be eliminated entirely, a 20 percent reduction in deaths due to cancer would result (based upon the assumption that 85 percent of lung cancer is causally related to cigarette smoking).

There is much evidence to suggest that many major diseases— lung cancer and heart disease, for instance—are often the direct result of 'abuses' of the body."[6]

Americans are literally killing themselves through "negative life-

---

[5]*Feeling Better, Doing Worse.*
[6]*Ibid.*

styles." Most people take illness for granted.

In *Whitmer's Guide to Total Wellness*, we are told that many of us, "have the attitude that illness is a part of living and each of us is allocated a certain amount." Bill Whitmer tells us, however, that we have the capability of either encouraging or preventing illness within our own lives.

First, we must avoid the "Five Deadly S's—smoking, sitting, snacks, sugar and salt." When this step is taken, one can reduce the risk factors of serious illness and think in terms of being well, rather than ill. The best way to combat serious disease is to prevent it from occurring in the first place.

New interest in personal health has been labeled by Whitmer as the "Wellness Renaissance." He concludes that,

> *"The Wellness Renaissance is based upon the discovery that the human body is one of the most responsive organisms on earth. It responds in direct proportion to how it is treated. The body which is abused, misused, and neglected, malfunctions more often and wears out faster. This means the body ages quicker and dies sooner. On the other hand, the body which is cared for and taken care, has less problems. It suffers less breakdowns and lasts longer. The aging process slows down and life-span increases. It's that simple."[7]*

Through proper eating habits, regular exercise programs, and the elimination of smoking, excessive alcohol intake, obesity, and stress management, Americans can, to a large extent, control their own health destiny. Better health is ours for the taking. It is a matter of choice.

Who Should Pay?

Should the non-abusers bear any responsibility to provide health care for those who bring their illnesses upon themselves? If someone continues to abuse his body, knowing the potential harmful effects of such abuses, has he anyone to blame but himself? Should he honestly expect someone else to pay the consequences? Isn't that asking the innocent to shoulder part of the blame?

Human beings are fundamentally tough resilient animals, marvelously made, most of the time capable of getting along quite well on

---

[7] R. William Whitmer, *Whitmer's Guide to Total Wellness* (Doubleday & Company, 1982).

their own. Bad nutritional status (of the too-much fat intake resulting in obesity type) can predispose the individual to heart attacks, strokes, cancer of the gastro-intestinal tract, diabetes, liver and gall bladder disease, degenerative arthritis of the hips, knees, and ankles, and injuries. It is estimated that 16 percent of Americans under the age of 30 years are obese, while eighty million Americans are 20 pounds or more over their ideal weight for their height, sex and age. [8]

Maybe, the time has come to get Americans in better shape for the "rebirth of America"—should that become the destiny we choose. Recent studies indicate that each 10 percent (about 15-20 pounds) reduction in body weight in men who are 35 to 50 years of age would decrease the incidence of coronary disease by 20 percent.

The high carbohydrate (fast-food) diet, which is so typical of the American lifestyle, increases the risks of acquiring diabetes and leads to dental caries (cavities).

Alcoholism is thought to be both a mental and physical disease. Following repetitive intake of alcohol, the body's computer becomes confused. It begins to think that alcohol is Vitamin B, which it knows it needs, in order to function properly. Once it is "programmed" in this manner, when alcohol is absent from the blood messages are sent to the brain by the body's cells, saying we want and need this material in order to carry out our duties. This phenomenon is called "dependency," and a similar thing happens with other drugs, nasal sprays, caffeine, and nicotine.

The body can be re-programmed within about one week, but the subconscious mind continues to send messages to the conscious mind that it wants and needs alcohol. The individual must be strong and choose to let the conscious mind prevail in order to lick alcoholism.

The excessive use of alcohol has become a medical and financial albatross, as well as a threat to public safety. At least one-half of all deaths and injuries due to automobile accidents in America are associated with the excessive use of alcohol.

Most cancers are thought to be either directly or indirectly dependent upon environmental factors. Carcinogens (cancer-provoking substances) are commonly found in the food and the drugs we digest, the air we breathe, the water we drink, the occupations we pursue, and the habits in which we indulge. Individual resistance provided by

---

[8]*Feeling Better, Doing Worse.*

one's own immune system explains why two people exposed to the same environmental factors handle disease differently.[9]

Sharing Responsibility

In order to improve and maintain "good health" in America we must place equal responsibility on the medical community, the consumers, and the producers and manufacturers of risk-provoking substances. Along with this responsibility we must adopt a substantial change in behavior and habits so that Americans will feel as strongly about the *responsibility* for good health as we currently do about our "right" to good health.

Coach Bryant had a philosophy that is worthy of mentioning. He said, "The first thing one has to do in order to guarantee victory is to keep from losing." We have been losing the battle against personal responsibility in this health care crisis.

How do we keep from losing the battle of health care?

If no one smokes cigarettes or consumes alcohol and everyone exercises regularly, maintains optimal weight on a low-fat, low refined-carbohydrate, high fiber-content diet, reduces stress by simplifying his or her life, obtains adequate rest and recreation, understood the needs of infants and children for the proper nutrition and nurturing of their intellectual and effective development, had available to them, and would use genetic counseling, drank fluorinated water, followed the doctor's orders for medicines and self-care once disease was detected, used available health services at the appropriate time for screening examinations and health education-preventive medicine programs, the savings to the country would be mammoth. Billions of dollars could be saved. Those dollars could be used effectively to reduce human misery, and help foster a significant improvement in the quality of life for all Americans. Our country would be strengthened immeasurably, and we could divert our human and financial energies to the other pressing issues of national and international concern.[10]

---

[9]*Ibid.*
[10]*Ibid.*

A Winning Plan

Now, we have examined the problem. We have also reviewed the solution. All that is left is the execution of the winning game plan. As is the case with an athletic team, each player must do his part in order to achieve a common goal. Earlier in this book, we explained that "oneness" is the feeling by individuals that they are an integral part of a whole; that by sacrificing individual glory they could help their teammates reach greater heights.

Rights vs Responsibilities

The recent emphasis in America has been on individual rights as contrasted to responsibilities, not unlike the athlete who wants all the glory and expects special privileges. There has been an erosion of the principles of individual responsibility and initiative which have made our nation great. Albert Schweitzer said, "man must cease attributing his problem to his environment, and learn again to exercise . . . his personal responsibility. . ."[11]

Unless we, as individual citizens, are willing to accept some of the responsibility, we should stop complaining about the steadily rising cost of health care. There is a clear choice: to change our personal abuses and bad habits or to stop complaining.

From the beginning of time, human beings have always valued good health. This value is, no doubt, based upon our survival instinct. While pursuing good health, man has resorted to practices ranging from witchcraft to exorcism and the supernatural. Only recently have knowledge, philosophy, and reason replaced these less civilized practices. Regardless of whether one believes that the source of good health is to be found in mysticism, religion, or science, what is important is the existence of good health itself. Without health, we lose sight of the many other things that are also important in our lives.

There is an Arabian Proverb which states, "He who has health, has hope; and he who has hope has everything."[12]

As we accept technological advances and look toward America's health care future, shouldn't the government and legal profession move back to their respective places and get out of emergency

---

[11]*Peter's Quotations* p. 452.
[12]*Treasury of Familiar Quotations* p. 122.

rooms, operating rooms, hospital wards, and doctors offices?

The *American Heritage Dictionary* defines "attorney at law" as "one who is qualified to represent clients in a court of law and to advise then on legal matters." Upon graduation, today's attorney receives the degree, Doctor of Jurisprudence. His "doctor's" degree appears to have taken on an expanded interpretation.

By using the current tort system, plaintiff attorneys have too much influence on how and by whom health care is provided. The ever present threat of medical malpractice suits certainly has contributed to increasing the cost of obtaining and providing health care. A similar problem exists throughout all sectors of the market place. Liability insurance premiums have skyrocketed for everyone. The medical and legal professions must work together to get things back in perspective.

When did the pendulum begin to swing too far? The founders of the Association of Trail Lawyers of America (ATLA) initiated what has been called a "Renaissance of Torts"—a kind of "declaration of independence" for plaintiffs. Since the establishment of the ATLA, the reported financial verdicts have risen from $50,000 (1948) to $4 million (1976) and on to a more recent $11 million verdict against a Mobile, Alabama surgeon in 1985.[13]

I don't believe it was meant for the legal profession to be on the field of play in the medical arena, certainly not to the extent which now exists. The current system allows the legal profession and their hired traveling physician witnesses (many of whom do not practice medicine) to treat every case with 20/20 hindsight. What America needs are prudent professionals with foresight. It appears that a need exists for a "Renaissance of Tort Reform." There is growing support within the legal profession to do just that.

May both sides, lawyers and non-lawyers draw upon wisdom, accept the challenge, and get on with it. The *system* needs reform. The destiny of Medicine and Law in America is a matter of choice! Let's huddle and make the commitment to do what must be done. America awaits the verdict.

---

[13]*My Learned Friends,* Cincinnati, Ohio: Anderson Publishing Company, 1976).

PART VI

THE MASTER PLAN

CHAPTER 25

YESTERDAY, TODAY AND TOMORROW

*"When I want to understand what is happening today or try
to decide what will happen tomorrow, I look back."*[1]

As I have "looked back" I realize that mankind has come full circle.
There are no new problems, no new answers, just different players.

One of Ralph Waldo Emerson's rural neighbors borrowed from
him a copy of the works of Plato. "Did you enjoy the book?" asked
Emerson when it was returned. "I did," replied the neighbor. "This
Plato has a lot of my ideas."

One of my goals in developing this book has been to demonstrate
how the ideas of learned and experienced men have been brought into
reality through the accomplishments and adversities encountered by
one man—not that my life has necessarily been more special than
any other. But I have studied and witnessed the endeavors of a few
great individuals in their pursuit of excellence. So far we have examined the accomplishments and adversities encountered by both individuals and groups because looking back at what has already
occurred gives us the insight needed to see the future.

---

[1]Oliver Wendell Holmes, Jr., *Peter's Quotations.*

Each of the greats understood human nature and knew how to deal with the unpredictability of man's behavior. Each kept life in perspective while enjoying achievements and combatting assaults. Each knew his own strengths and weaknesses and worked within his limitations with purpose and conviction. Let's face it, we're not talking about ghosts, myths, or illusions, we are talking about reality—real people—people who transcended mediocrity due to commitment to excellence. We keep their wisdom alive when we follow their teachings.

What makes man unique? It is his ability to reason that distinguishes him from other species. The human brain is a unique type of computer afforded with the capability of dealing in facts, probabilities, and illusions—the ability to project an image that does not yet exist. In his individuality, man has certain predictable characteristics called behavior, some inbred, some learned. Each member of the species is a product of both genetics and environment. Both are important. Since our pre-natal period, information has been fed into our human computer, cataloged, and stored for retrieval.

Life is like a game of chess. While jumbled together in a box, no one piece possesses any distinction or power over the other. Not until the characters are removed from storage and placed in their respective positions on the chessboard is any meaning given to their individuality.

While the game is on we learn to deal with the contrasting power of queens and pawns, to be on the alert for the cunning moves of knights, to respect that for which the bishops stand, to dream of owning castles, and to guard our kings against those who would assault them.

In the real world the data we use to develop our plan of attack, or defense, originates from our environment, how we respond to our environment is, in part, based upon our genetics and how we are programmed. Tampering with the mind is an art, science, and business. It can be, and is, done in many ways. Alcohol, drugs, and certain chemicals can affect neural responses, and alter behavior and performance. Brainwashing (a kind of re-programming) can modify attitudes and convictions.

Propaganda is a more subtle form of brainwashing. It's all around us. Humans are bombarded with slanted information about products, services, and ideologies through well-conceived advertising and promotional campaigns. Today, with television, radio, movies, and the print media, it is easier to recast the minds of the adult public and mold the minds of youth. As a result of seeing the movie, "Ice Castles," Chanee (our daughter) became obsessed with ice skating. For six years, our family's lifestyle changed so that she could pursue her dream. It is bothersome to know that a movie could effect a child to the extent this one did. Fortunately, this particular movie had a *positive* effect. What about some of the things to which our children are exposed? The subconscious mind never forgets what it has seen, or heard. That input is stored in the memory bank.

The capacity and potential efficiency of our human "computer" is most likely inherited, but the quality of material retrieved can be no better than what has been fed into it. That's why environment becomes such an important factor in our development.

The subconscious mind makes no distinction between good and bad material. It stores all information. The super-ego or conscience either suppresses or retrieves the information it needs to deal with any situation. As we learn more about the relationship between chemical imbalances within the central nervous system and altered behavior, scientists may eventually be able to control emotion and intelligence.

Unlike a mechanical computer, repetition is a more important factor with respect to learned behavior.

People often react to stimuli in a manner similar to Pavlov's dog. When the insecure man hears the bell of success being tolled for his colleague, his most common response is jealousy. The sound of someone else's success triggers a conditioned response. He salivates too, but the stiumlus is envy. To reach a homeostatic state the insecure man generally tries to slow the pace to his own level of incompetence, but he has another choice. He could also choose to pick himself up, establish a goal, develop a plan, and climb upon "the shoulders of giants" leaving mediocrity behind—to modify or recast his behavior. That's what the achievers do.

Adaptation is one characteristic which all humans possess. People can be "programmed." That's why environment is so important during development. Because a child's mind is a precious commodity, thoughtful parents should control what his computer is exposed to and feed it with positive thoughts, especially during the formative years. Prepare your children for life's challenges.

Upon reaching adulthood, we should have learned to distinguish between good and evil, be equipped to establish our own goals and values, and be able to modify our behavior accordingly. If we can do this, we can achieve victory over shortcomings and step over roadblocks along the road to success.

Life is Short

Leaving things to chance allows opportunity to pass by. There was a sign on the wall of my high school football dressing room which stated, "Luck is what happens when preparation meets opportunity." Simply waiting around for something to happen until we reach some magical age in our lives invites disappointment or failure. We never know how long our journey will last, therefore, we need to make every minute count.

Dr. Charles Allen tells the story about a woman who took her first journey on a train.

> As soon as she reached her seat, she began fumbling with the window to be sure that she got exactly the right amount of air. Then she pulled the window shade up and down until she got exactly the right amount of light coming in. Then she worked with her baggage to get it placed just right. Then she took off her hat and was very careful to put it where it would not get smashed. Then she took her mirror and comb and combed her hair to be sure it was just right. Just about the time she got everything fixed and settled down comfortably, the conductor called out her station. As she got off the train she said, "If I had known the trip was going to be so short, I would not have fussed so much over unimportant details!"[2]

Life is a short train ride. Dr. Allen reminds us that many of the details we fuss over throughout our lives are not worth it. When we realize how short life is, there are many things that are *un*important in the long run. Things that really matter are often neglected or put off until the ride is nearly over. It's not always what a person did, but what he doesn't do that plagues him.

---

[2]Dr. Charles Allen, *We Are Never Alone.*

What Is Man?

Mark Twain was a man who possessed great insight. In "What Is Man," he wrote: "The fact that man knows right from wrong proves his *intellectual* superiority to the other creatures; but the fact that he can do wrong proves his *moral* inferiority to any other creature."

To overcome the inherent weakness of our species and achieve victory over shortcomings, we could choose to latch on to the wisdom of those greats who have shown us the way in our pursuit of excellence. This is the main reason this book has been written—to share what I have learned through my personal experiences with many of them and through their writings. No one can accomplish great things without the help of others.

I have reviewed personal accomplishments and challenges only to demonstrate how the lessons I learned from my role models can be applied to everyday life and to demonstrate that accomplishments and adversities go hand and hand.

Since I was old enough to realize that others knew what I wanted to know, I have attempted to feed my "computer" with what has already been proven to work. I continue to search for answers to one of man's challenges—being the best he can be through prosperity and adversity. While looking for answers, it is important to balance the good and bad. . .

> *"Success is never final and failure never fatal. It's courage that counts."*[3]

Self-analysis and self-esteem are the keys to self-control. The secret of survival is in knowing one's strengths and weaknesses, then realizing how far he can be pushed. The first step in getting better however, is to be honest with oneself. When the problem is defined, it is 90 per cent solved. Once the good qualities are identified, we build upon them. No matter how insignificant one might feel when he sets out to do what needs to be done, he should never underestimate his potential.

> *"A handful of pine seed will cover mountains with the green majesty of a forest."*[4]

---

[3]George Tilden, *Seeds To Sow* p. 28.
[4]William Sharp, *Seeds To Sow* p. XII.

The Creation

But, what about this creature man? How does he fit into the master plan? From whence did he come? Furthermore, where is he going? Since Eden, he has been created imperfect. He acquires other faults along the way, but he also has the potential for greatness. How and why did man become the vehicle through which wisdom travels through time?

In many respects humans are superior to other animals, however, keener senses and greater endurance can be found throughout the animal kingdom. The dog has superior smell, the eagle superior sight, the deer superior hearing, the horse and mule greater endurance.

This is not the appropriate forum to debate evolution and creation, but there are some interesting questions. Is it possible that the end product (man) may have been created by a combination of both? As long as God was responsible, how He did it is irrelevant except that it is part of the master plan that man wants to understand.

Darwin's theory of evolution is based on a complex process in which life supposedly originated as a single cell formed by an accident of nature in a pool of water. He concluded that from this one cell, over millions of years all living creatures have evolved.

There is enough biological similarity of the various species to support some of the more *advanced* portions of the theory of evolution.

Recent archeological finds suggest that the earliest forms of man may have existed around Lake Turkana in Kenya, Africa. Skeletons of various ape species have been found along side the skeletal remains of what appears to be the earliest man, suggesting a close environmental and biological relationship. One only needs to study comparative anatomy to recognize the biological and physiological relationship which clearly exists between the various species of animals and see how such an evolutionary theory could be used to explain *part* of the Creation.

People whose ancestoral roots sprang from inhabitants of geographical regions with sunny climates inherit dark or black skin. This physical characteristic may have evolved out of necessity to protect them from the sun's damaging ray. Others, whose forebearers inhabited geographic regions, where the sun rarely shines, inherit white skin. If all men sprang from Adam, was it the ability to evolve or adapt to environment that explains differing physical characteristics within the same species? How else do we explain the existence of black, white, red, brown and yellow skin within a single species from a common origin?

The late Herbert W. Armstrong in his "Plain Truth" magazine stated that,

> "evolution is the agnostic's or atheist's attempted explanation of the presence of a creation *without* the pre-existence of an intelligent creator."

The Bible tells us that man was created by God "in His own image on the sixth day" from the dust of the earth.

How then, could both "theories" have validity? Is it possible that some of the evolutionary events postulated by Darwin could have occurred under the direction of the "Intelligent Creator?"

Today, embryo implantations are being performed in medical centers throughout the world. Could this "technological breakthrough" be a revelation to mankind by the "Intelligent Creator?" Is embryo implantation the missing link?

The puzzle is certainly complex. At this point in time, we do not have all of the answers. Maybe we never will. The answers lie beyond science. What about that photograph of the UFO?

As our knowledge of man and the universe increases, one day we may be able to better understand the planned relationship between man and his brother, and man and his Creator. On a recent program about early mankind on the Public Broadcasting System, it was said that, "Mankind is a single species with a common origin and a common destiny."

At the time mankind develops common goals and common understanding, he may then realize what that "destiny" is. I believe that great men and women (giants) are placed on earth to show us the way, to disseminate knowledge and wisdom.

CHAPTER 26

"THE SELECTION OF WISDOM"

As we have seen, few things are new. Others have experienced situations similar to what confronts us. We can gain wisdom from the experiences of those who have already felt the heat of the fire. When it comes to events that involve people and their behavior, we, more than likely, discover what others have known for centuries. Remember, we can learn by trial and error or from drawing upon the wisdom of those who already know the answers.

From examining our past experiences, each of us eventually reaches some conclusions about ourselves (self-image), our fellow man, and the rest of the world. Along the way we usually adopt a philosophy or creed by which we respond to events and individuals (self-control).

An Ace to Keep

In the next few pages, I will attempt to "package" the philosophy I have adopted from the words and deeds of wise and great teachers. This synopsis may become an "ace that you can keep," too.

Bergen Evens has said, "wisdom is meaningless until your own experience has given it meaning... and there is wisdom in the selection of wisdom."[1]

---

[1]*Peter's Quotations.*

I believe in the selection of wise role models.

No one is more blind than he who has the capacity of vision and simply refuses to see. The bookshelves of the world are filled with the wisdom of wise and excellent men and women. Their teachings, however, do not leap off the pages and into our heads. In order to acquire wisdom, one must search for it. In order to achieve excellence, one must pursue it. Vicariously, we can live the lives of great individuals through the experiences they've recorded. Throughout this book winning game plans have been shared. Good times and bad have been revealed. Both are a necessary part of man's struggle to find fulfillment. An individual seeking victory must be committed to deal with the challenges he is bound to face.

In my quest to live out a dream to become the best facial surgeon I could be, I have taken some direct hits from detractors casting stones. As a child, I was taught that "sticks and stones may break my bones, but words will never hurt me." The author of those lines must never have been the victim of an attempted character assassination. Slander hurts, too.

Rudyard Kipling's "If" offers advice during times of difficulty. "If" provides the solution to almost any challenge that one could encounter. By understanding the message contained within its lines, one can view his problems in a more mature manner, put difficult situations into perspective, and respond to challenges with better insight. With some poetic license, I have "updated" the language and given it a bit of personal interpretation. My "If" is entitled, "Say Yes." In it are the keys to controlling one's destiny.

SAY YES!

Will you keep your head when others are losing theirs—
    Campaigning with malice against you?
Will you trust yourself when others doubt you,
    But be tolerant of their doubting too?
Will you be patient and not be tired by waiting?
    When you're lied about, will your life prove them lies?
When being hated, will you rise above those hating;
    And yet—don't look too good, nor talk too wise?

Will you dream—yet not make dreams your master;
   Will you think—but make work your aim?
When life deals either Triumph or Disaster
   Will you treat those two just the same?
Will you stand to hear the truth being
   Twisted to make you look a fool;
Or watch all the things you gave your life to, broken,
   Then build again with battered tools?
Will you put at stake the things you've longed for
   And risk a chance to be "the best,"
Then lose, and start a new beginning;
   Plan next time to pass life's test?
Will you make your heart and mind defend you
   After they feel they've reached the end?

     . . . .

If you will "say yes" to all these things. . .
   And then,
Hold on when there is nothing left within you
   Except a voice which cries: "You will not bend,"
Yours is the Earth and all that's in it,
   A fate of choice is yours, my friend.

Trying to follow Kipling's package of wisdom and using the insight that I have gained from great minds, I adopted a philosophy of life which has now been shared with all who have read this book. With syllogistic reasoning as a foundation, I recognized from whence I came, what factors allowed me to arrive at this point in my life, where I am going from here, and how I plan to get there.

John Ruskin has written, "The greatest thing a human soul ever does in this world is to *see* something and tell what he *saw* in a plain way. . . To see clearly is poetry, prophecy and religion all in one."[2]

I have told what I have seen, and tried to tell it in a plain way. I hope my efforts will help some other person who has a dream to "load" his

---

[2]George Seldes, "Modern Painters," *The Great Thoughts* p. 360.

(or her) wagon so that they will be better prepared for what lies ahead for them.

Through the eyes of those wiser than I, I have had the opportunity to see things I might otherwise have never seen and to seek solutions to problems some fear to challenge. I have been afforded chances, made some choices, and accepted the challenges. Through self-analysis, I learned who I am and realized my limitations. I plan to face what lies ahead with realistic expectations. As I set my sail toward new horizons, I hope that "God (will) grant me the serenity to accept the things I cannot change, the courage to change the things I can, and the wisdom to know the difference."[3]

Serenity comes from self-analysis, courage from self-esteem. Wisdom is acquired by following in the footsteps of great people.

When I am confronted by a challenge and I want to know how the great men and women might respond, I look back, develop a plan, then forge ahead knowing it is possible to transcend mediocrity. I've seen that philosophy work for others who have pursued and achieved excellence.

The Rewards

As the two of them looked back over one great man's pursuit of excellence, St. Peter probably said to Coach Bryant,

> *"They say you were the best*
> *At molding young boys into men,*
> *The best at teaching leadership,*
> *And teaching how to win.*
> *They say you taught with discipline,*
> *Of struggle and of strife,*
> *And helped a lot of young men*
> *Cross that great goal line of life."*

To which Coach Bryant might have replied,

> *"The only thing I wanted*
> *Was for them to understand*

---

[3]Anonymous.

That by believing in themselves,
They'd be a better man.
It wasn't the winning or the losing,
Glamour or the fame
It's what they were that was important,
And how they played the game."
                    ("St. Peter and the Bear," Lee Cooper, 1983)

And then as he walked through "The Gates" and looked around him, Coach Bryant might have added, *"The price of victory is high—but so are the rewards."*

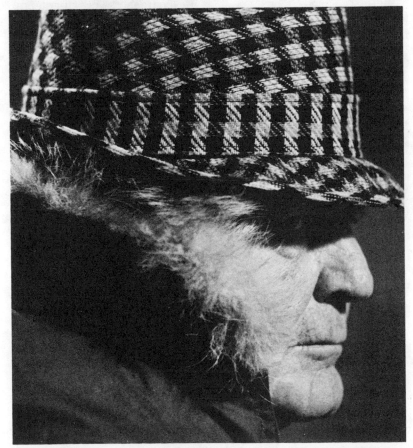

"The only thing I wanted was for them to understand that by believing in themselves, they'd be a better man." (Coach Paul "Bear" Bryant)

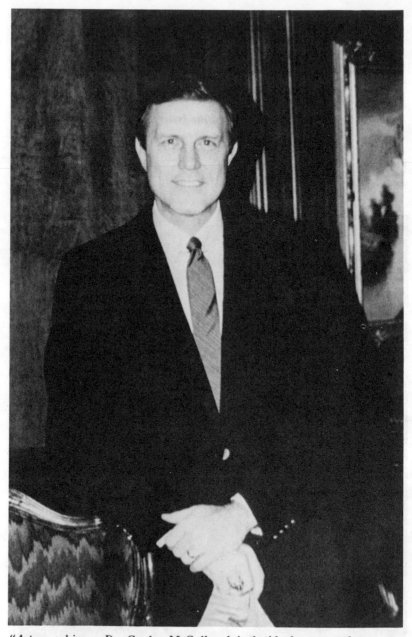

"A true achiever, Dr. Gaylon McCollough is the ideal person to have written this introspective, stimulating book."
    Fred Russell, Vice President, Nashville Banner, Nashville, Tennessee

Throughout this book I have attempted to credit those responsible for preserving the sayings of wise and excellent men and women. The great ones of yesterday and today lift the rest of us up with their knowledge, preserve us with their courage, and sustain us with their wisdom. Their standards, convictions, and methods of problem solving can live again if adopted by others.

What we have seen, we owe to giants. Where we go and what we choose to become is up to us. Destiny is a "thing to be achieved." A course pursuing excellence is a matter of choice. Victory over mediocrity is obtainable for anyone willing to pay the price. Climb upon the "shoulders of giants." See the price and rewards of victory.

There are things yet to do—chances, choices, and challenges—mountains yet to conquer. The expedition is far from being over. The keys to reaching the summit must be self-analysis, self-esteem, and self-control. Each person can make his choice.

Whenever we question our capabilities, we might remember that: "There is a kind of greatness which does not depend upon fortune . . . *it is the value we set upon ourselves* . . . and it is this which commonly raises us more above other men than birth, rank or even merit itself."[4]

First and Ten

There are scores of individuals with more intelligence, wisdom and talent than I; however, I have a chance to be a player in life's game. I choose to play on the team coached by giants.

> *"I am only one, but I am one. I cannot do everything, but I can do something. What I can do, I should do, and with the help of God, (*and the giants*) I will do . . .*[5] what I can do.

This game "ain't" over, not yet . . . it's first and ten . . . huddle up . . .

---

[4]La Rochefoucauld, *Treasury of Familiar Quotations* p. 54.
[5]Everett Hale, *The Rebirth of America* p. 223.